CAUSE, DISEASE AND EFFECT PHENOMENA
FUNDAMENTAL ASPECTS OF HOMOEOPATHY

CAUSE, DISEASE AND EFFECT PHENOMENA
FUNDAMENTAL ASPECTS OF HOMOEOPATHY

Dr. RANJIT K. ROY

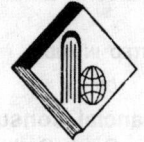

B. JAIN PUBLISHERS (P) LTD.

NOTE FROM THE PUBLISHERS

Any information given in this book is not intended to be taken as a replacement for medical advice. Any person with a condition requiring medical attention should consult a qualified practitioner or therapist.

© All rights are reserved

No part of this publication may be reproduced, stored in a retrieval system or transmitted, in any form or by any means, mechanical, photocopying, recording or otherwise, without prior written permission of the publishers.

First Edition : November 2001

Price: Rs. 75.00

Published by

Kuldeep Jain

for

B. Jain Publishers (P) Ltd.

1921, Chuna Mandi, St. 10th Paharganj,
New Delhi-110 055
Ph: 3670430, 3670572, 3683200, 3683300
Fax: 011-3610471 & 3683400
Website: www.bjainbooks.com, Email: bjain@vsnl.com

PRINTED IN INDIA
by
Unisons Techno Financial Consultants (P) Ltd.
522, FIE, Patpar Ganj, Delhi-110 092

ISBN : 81-7021-1093-5
BOOK CODE : BR-5504

Dedication

This book is dedicated to all those who worked incessantly and immensely to develop homoeopathy into an outstanding therapeutic system to treat, manage and cure diseases to alleviate human sufferings.

Acknowledgements

Through the *Organon of medicine,* Master Hahnemann presented to the world humanity a completely new healing system and a new field of medicine. The work of the Organon is simply outstanding, infallible and mind-boggling. No words, written or talked, are rich enough to pay a right tribute to Dr. Hahnemann, a great master-mind and physician of the nineteenth century.

During my endeavour to write this book, I received a lot of inspiration and support from my family members: my wife and two children. The manuscript of the book was computer-processed by Mr. M. H. Rizvi whom I thank in abundance. I sincerely thank the Publishing House, B. Jain Publishers (P) Ltd., New Delhi, for bringing out the book in a time-bound schedule.

Prologue

The subject of Homoeopathy is very vast. Master Hahnemann introduced this subject as a healing art in the year 1796. Since then it has grown over the last 200 years. Now its volume is stupendous. In spite of its vastness, homoeopathy has three main component parts. These are the *Organon of Medicine,* the *Materia Medica* and *Repertory.* The Organon provides us the main principles of homoeopathic methodologies. The Materia Medica presents us the medicinal symptomatologies and the Repertory does the classification of symptoms. Both Materia Medica and Repertory are used for working procedures to select simillimum. The Materia Medica was formed from the provings of medicines and clinical experiences. The Repertory is a unique structure of individual symptoms of the Materia Medica, organised systematically, under various broad and minor rubrics. A lot of further work are seen on the Materia Medica and Repertory. On the other hand, further work on the Organon have been rather limited although there is equally great scope to work on the Organon.

The importance of the Organon is that it is the main foundation of homoeopathy as a healing science. Every para of the Organon has its deep meaning, values and implications.

certain molecular biological entities/events. Such efforts to integrate molecular biology into homoeopathy from various angles can be a good step and beneficial for greater understanding of many homoeopathic events. In short, this book shall benefit many of the students, researchers and practitioners in the field of homoeopathy.

Dated : 30*th* October, 2001
Place : Kohima

Dr. P. Savino
Registrar
Board of Homoeopathic
System of Medicine,
Nagaland

Foreword

New data, concepts, ideas, analysis, interpretation, evaluation and synthesis are constantly enriching the field of homoeopathic therapeutics. This book on *'cause, disease and effect phenomena'* by Dr. Ranjit K. Roy also presents before us some new ideas and ways of considering, evaluating and interpreting human diseases and making strategies for their treatment. Method of splitting a human sickness into three clear-cut component phenomena and evaluating each phenomenon in its own worth is an innovative idea. It looks very systematic, logical and scientific. Practically, all homoeopathic methodologies work on these three spheres of symptoms, though not clearly distinguished at present. Differentiating the effect phenomenon of a disesase is a new element introduced by the author into the aspect of remedy selection. It is actually the cause, disease and effect symptoms which represent a Hahnemannian Totality. Inclusion of human constitution and miasm in the category of causative phenomenon can play a vital role in disease evaluation and treatment strategy as emphasized by the author. It is also quite revealing that the author attempted to relate some of the homoeopathic phenomena (e.g. miasm and constitution) to

But it is almost forgotten by the most neophytes of homoeopathy after formal education. Homoeopathic methodologies cannot progress leaving the work of Organon in the backyard. The Organon, a core of homoeopathy, needs to be worked out and expanded further along with the Materia Medica and Repertory for overall progress of homoeopathic therapeutics. This book is a preliminary effort to work on a few aspects of the Organon which Master Hahnemann experienced, visualised and discussed particularly about diseases, causations, constitutions and miasms. His valuable directions, ideas, concepts, experiences and methodologies are depicted in various paragraphs of the Organon.

Due to intricate and disseminated nature of the information spread over the whole of Organon, the students of homoeopathy particularly the neophytes often face dilemas in clearly conceiving some of the essences of remedy evaluation. It is in this context that I attempted some efforts to analyse and systematise a few aspects of the Organon. What I could observe from Master Hahnemann's discourse through the Organon is that a human sickness is constituted of and can be split into three distinct component phenomena. These are which I described as *'causative phenomenon'*, *'disease phenomenon'* and *'effect phenomenon'* of a human sickness. These are three most fundamental aspects of homoeopathy on which the paradigm of remedy selection can be based. The spectrum of totality of symptoms or essences or characteristic (peculiar) symptoms, all actually belong to these above three categories of phenomena. This way of considering basic spheres of symptoms and an understanding of a human sickness on these terms can probably add to homoeopathy another strong foundation as a healing science. The collection, analysis and evaluation of symptoms — all generally proceed from this structured foundation.

Mixing up of all categories of symptoms at random probably makes the selection methodology of totality more complex and confounded, particularly to the most neophytes. The concept of *cause, disease and effect phenomena* of a human sickness is a scientific fact and systematically provides at the fundamental level a very logical and scientific basis for further work on an important aspect of homoeopathic therapeutics, the selection of remedies.

Place : Dimapur – 797112
Date: 28th September, 2001 *Ranjit K. Roy*

QUOTATION

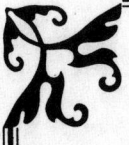 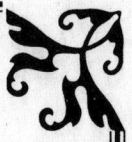

" EGO IS A DELUSION, ...
TRANSCEND THESE AND

YOU WILL REACH THE HIGHEST LEVEL OF
SPIRITUALITY"

Dr. Rajan Sankaran
INDIA

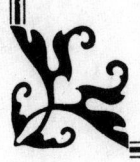 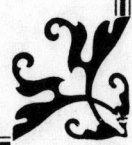

QUOTATION

"......... EGO IS A DELUSION, ...
TRANSCEND THIS AND
YOU WILL REACH THE HIGHEST LEVEL OF
SPIRITUALITY"

Dr. Rajesh Sankaran
INDIA

Contents

ACKNOWLEDGEMENTS xiii
FOREWORD xiv
PROLOGUE xvi

1. HUMAN DISEASES 1

1.1 Disease-causing Agents 1

1.1.1 Biological agents 2

1.1.2 Non-biological agents 2

1.1.2.1 Physical agents 2

1.1.2.2 Chemical agents 2

1.1.2.2.1 Endogenous chemical agents 2

1.1.2.2.2 Exogenous chemical agents 3

1.1.2.3 Mechanical agents 3

1.1.2.4 Nutritive agents 3

1.2. Types of diseases 4

1.2.1 Congenital diseases 4

1.2.1.1 Diseases of gene mutations 4

1.2.1.2 Diseases of chromosomal mutations 4

1.2.1.3 Diseases caused by environmental factors 4

1.2.2 Acquired diseases 4

1.2.2.1 Communicable diseases 5

1.2.2.1.1 Bacterial diseases 5

1.2.2.1.2 Viral diseases 5

1.2.2.1.3 Protozoan diseases 5

1.2.2.1.4 Fungal diseases 5

1.2.2.1.5 Helminth diseases 6

1.2.2.1.6 Rickettsial diseases 6

1.2.2.1.7 Spirochaetal diseases 6

1.2.2.1.8 Contagious diseases 6

1.2.2.1.9 Non-contagious diseases 6

1.2.2.1.9.1 Deficiency diseases 6

1.2.2.1.9.2 Degenerative diseases 7

1.2.2.1.9.3 Allergic diseases 7

1.2.2.1.9.4 Cancerous diseases 7

1.3 Occupational diseases 8

1.4 AIDS And Homoeopathic Medicines 8

1.5 Remarks 11

2. BACKGROUND METHODOLOGIES IN HOMOEOPATHY 13

2.1 Hahnemannian totality 14

2.2 Kent's constitution 15

2.3 Boenninghausen's grand symptom 18

2.4 Hering's law of cure 20

2.5 George Vithoulkas' essences 23

2.6 Jan Scholten's Group analysis 25

2.7 Rajan Sankaran's methods of delusion, central disturbance and situational materia medica 27

2.8 Thematic determination of cancer remedies 29

2.9 Recognition of certain problems 34

3. CONCEPTUALISATION 37

3.1 The concept evolution 37

3.2 Cause 39

3.2 Disease 39

3.4 Effect 40

3.5 Two types of mentals 44

3.6 Three dynamic phenomena 44

3.7 Synthesis 45

4. FIVE OUTSTANDING CASE STUDIES **49**

4.1 Chronic bodyache 49

4.2 Epilepsy 51

4.3 Chronic appendicitis 51

4.4 Panic attack 52

4.5 Sudden fever 53

5. CAUSATIVE PHENOMENON **55**

5.1 Two types 55

5.2 Cheek-bone tumor 56

5.3 Ganglion 56

5.4 Sciatica 57

5.5 Mental depression 57

5.6 Cerebral stroke 58

5.7 Coccyx pain 59

5.8 High fever 59

5.9 Excessive vomiting 60

5.10 Shoulder rheumatism 60

5.11 Diarrhea/dysentery 61

5.12 Some important causative remedies 61

6. MIASM AS A CAUSATIVE PHENOMENON 65

6.1 The concept 65

6.2 Significance 66

6.3 Miasmatic symptoms 67

6.4 Miasmatic applications 69

6.5 Some Case Reports 70

6.5.1 Asthmatic bronchitis 70

6.5.2 Leucorrhea 71

6.5.3 Chronic sinusitis 71

6.5.4 Venereal disease 72

6.5.6 Chronic tonsillitis 72

6.5.7 Down's syndrome 73

6.6 Where to use miasmatic remedies 74

6.7 Background miasm and Disease miasm 75

7. CONSTITUTIONAL SUSCEPTIBILITY AS A CAUSATIVE PHENOMENON 79

7.1 The concept 79

7.2 Few constitutional remedies and their characteristics 81

7.3 Remarks 82

7.4 Some Case Reports 83
7.4.1 Hydatid cyst 83
7.4.2 Appendicitis 84
7.4.3 Diabetes mellitus 85
7.4.4 Epilepsy 86
7.4.5 Leucorrhea 87
7.4.6 Hypertension 88
7.4.7 Peptic ulcer 89
7.4.8 Unhealthy growth of hair 89
7.5 Where to use constitutional remedies 91

8. DISEASE PHENOMENON 93
8.1 The Meaning 93
8.2 Some Case Reports 94
8.2.1 Chronic backache 94
8.2.2 Low back pain 95
8.2.3 Nose bleeding 95
8.2.4 Respiratory difficulty 96
8.2.5 Right-sided hernia 96
8.2.6 Intermittent fever 97

8.2.7 Knee pain 97

8.2.8 Hernia 97

8.2.9 Coughing, fever and hemoptysis 98

8.3 Remarks 98

9. EFFECT PHENOMENON 101

9.1 The symptom evolution 101

9.2 A subtle differentiation 102

9.3 Discussion 104

9.4 Some Case Reports 105

9.4.1 Tongue ulceration 105

9.4.2 Pharyngitis-tonsillitis 106

9.4.3 Breast nodules 106

9.4.4 Chronic gastric trouble 107

9.4.5 Chronic colitis 108

9.4.6 Chronic renal failure 108

9.4.7 Hypertension 109

9.4.8 Pancreatic cancer 110

9.4.9 Diabetes mellitus 110

9.4.10 Fish bone injury 111

9.5 Remarks 112

10. GENES AND MIASMS 115

10.1 Heredity and DNA 115

10.2 Genes and Environment 116

10.3 Human variations and Mutations 117

10.4 Miasmatic doctrine of Hahnemann 117

10.5 Miasmatic susceptibilities 118

10.6 Induced mutation: An example of environmental interaction 120

10.7 Inherited miasms and Acquired miasms 122

10.8 Gene expressions and Homoeopathic constitutions . 123

10.9 Genotype/Phenotype and their implications in remedy selection 124

10.10 Dominant and recessive characters of genes and their implications in homoeopathy 125

10.11 Remarks 126

11. SPEED OF SYMPTOM EVOLUTION AND ITS IMPLICATIONS 129

11.1 Some tenets of law 129

11.2 The case report 130

11.3 Analysis of the case 131

11.4 Synthesis 132

12. TYPES AND NATURE OF MEDICINAL AGGRAVATIONS 135

12.1 Aphorism 157 and 158 135

12.2 Three case reports 136

12.3 Analyses of the cases 137

12.4 Discussion 139

13. DISEASE VERSUS MIND: A HOMOEOPATHIC UNDERSTANDING 141

14. RELATIVE FREQUENCY OF MANIFESTATIONS OF CDE (CAUSE-DISEASE-EFFECT) PHENOMENA ... 147

15. RELATIVE IMPORTANCE OF CDE PHENOMENA 151

15.1 Background 151

15.2 Limitations 152

15.3 Some case examples 153

15.3.1 Allergic itching 153

15.3.2 Eczema 154

15.3.3 Excessive hair fall 154

15.4 Remarks 155

16. EPILOGUE **157**
BIBLIOGRAPHY **165**

CHAPTER-1

Human Diseases

To discuss about human diseases, it is necessary to consider what is health at a first instance. According to the definition of the World Health Organisation (WHO), *health is a state of perfect physical, mental and social well being.* It is a state of human body when all its systems and organs function appropriately. Thus, a complete harmony is maintained between the body and the environment. So, any situation/condition that can interfere with or impair the normal functioning of the body can be called a disease. In homoeopathy, Master Hahnemann considered a disease to be a sickness of the body, mind and emotion. Thus, any condition that could alter the normal state of body, mind and emotion was considered as a disease/disorder. We recapitulate here in brief the various types of human diseases and their causative agents.

1.1 DISEASE-CAUSING AGENTS

The substances which have capacity to cause human diseases are called disease agents. These are mainly of two types i.e. biological and non-biological.

1.1.1 BIOLOGICAL AGENTS

These are some micro-organisms which enter the human body from outside environment, multiply and then cause infectious diseases. They include bacteria, virus, fungus, protozoan, helminth, etc. Some of the infectious diseases, for example, are tuberculosis, typhoid, hepatitis, pneumonia, measles, chicken pox, etc.

1.1.2 NON-BIOLOGICAL AGENTS

These can be classified into the following four types:—

1.1.2.1 PHYSICAL AGENTS

Some examples of physical agents are Sun light, heat, cold, humidity, nuclear radiations, x-rays, ultraviolet rays, electricity, sound, etc. The nuclear radiations, x-rays, ultraviolet rays, etc., have capacity to cause cancer. Excessive Sun burn can cause skin cancer (e.g. melanoma). Excess of humidity can predispose one to attacks of bronchial asthma.

1.1.2.2 CHEMICAL AGENTS

These can again be classified into two types i.e. endogenous and exogenous.

1.1.2.2.1 ENDOGENOUS CHEMICAL AGENTS

These substances are formed inside the human body. Some examples are hormones, enzymes, uric acid, insulin, thyroxin, cholesterol, etc. Excess of uric acid can cause gout. Excessive cholesterol can cause heart diseases. Deficiency of insulin can cause diabetes mellitus.

1.1.2.2.2 EXOGENOUS CHEMICAL AGENTS

These substances enter the human body from the surrounding environment through inhalation, ingestion or transfusion. Some examples are pollutants (e.g. NO_2, CO_2, CO, SO_2, vehicle emissions, dusts, metals), some allergens, polycyclic aromatic hydrocarbons, etc. Allergens can cause rhinitis, asthma, etc. Benzene can cause leukemia (blood cancer).

1.1.2.3 MECHANICAL AGENTS

These are mechanical shocks. Some examples are traumatic injuries, sprains, dislocations, fractures, etc. Physical sprain may indicate homoeopathic remedy *Arnica*. A needle injury may indicate *Ledum*. Injury of nerves may indicate Hypericum. Lacerated wounds may indicate *Calendula*.

1.1.2.4 NUTRITIVE AGENTS

Excesses or deficiencies of these substances can cause diseases. These agents are minerals, vitamins, fats, proteins, carbohydrates, water, etc. Deficiency of vitamin C can cause scurvy, that of D can cause rickets, that of A can cause night-blindness, etc. Deficiency of minerals like iron can cause anemia, that of iodine can cause goitre, that of fluorine can cause dental caries, etc. Excessive consumption of fat can cause gall bladder calculi, overweight, heart diseases and even cancer.

1.2. TYPES OF DISEASES

Depending on the incidences of diseases before or after birth, they are classified into two types i.e. congenital and acquired.

1.2.1 CONGENITAL DISEASES

These are diseases which are incident right from the time of birth. These are usually some anatomical or physiological defects. These are inherited and caused due to some kinds of gene/chromosomal defects or mutations.

1.2.1.1 DISEASES OF GENE MUTATIONS

Some examples are hemophilia, sickle cell anemia, albinism, color blindness, etc.

1.2.1.2 DISEASES OF CHROMOSOMAL MUTATIONS

Some examples are Down's syndrome, Turner's syndrome (in female), Klinefelter's syndrome (in male), etc.

1.2.1.3 DISEASES CAUSED BY ENVIRONMENTAL FACTORS

Some examples are cleft palate, hare lip, etc.

1.2.2 ACQUIRED DISEASES

These are diseases which are acquired after birth due to some causative agents which may be pathogenic or non-pathogenic. Depending upon the nature of transmission, these diseases are again classified into two types i.e. communicable diseases and non-communicable diseases.

1.2.2.1 COMMUNICABLE DISEASES

These are also called infectious diseases which can be transmitted from infected persons to healthy persons. These diseases are caused by some micro-organisms e.g. bacteria, virus, etc. The infectious diseases together are the leading cause of human death all over the world. Based on the nature of communicable diseases, they are further classified into the following types:—

1.2.2.1.1 BACTERIAL DISEASES
These are caused by bacterial infections. Some examples are tuberculosis, cholera, typhoid, tetanus, meningitis, diptheria, etc.

1.2.2.1.2 VIRAL DISEASES
These are caused by viral infections. Some examples are polio, chicken pox, small pox, measles, mumps, rabis, etc.

1.2.2.1.3 PROTOZOAN DISEASES
Some examples are malaria, amebiasis, Kala azar, etc.

1.2.2.1.4 FUNGAL DISEASES
Some examples are ringworm, athlete's foot, etc.

1.2.2.1.5 HELMINTH DISEASES

Some examples are ascariasis (caused by round worm), filariasis, trichinosis, taeniasis (caused by tape worm), etc.

1.2.2.1.6 RICKETTSIAL DISEASES

Some examples are typhus fever, trench fever, Rocky mountain fever, etc.

1.2.2.1.7 SPIROCHAETAL DISEASES

Some examples are syphilis, etc. Further, depending upon the mode of transmission of communicable diseases, they are classified into two types i.e. contagious and non-contagious diseases.

1.2.2.1.8 CONTAGIOUS DISEASES

These are diseases which can spread from an infected person to a healthy person by contact mechanism. Some examples are small pox, measles, leprosy, STD (sexually transmitted disease), etc.

1.2.2.1.9 NON-CONTAGIOUS DISEASES

These diseases do not spread from an infected person to a healthy person. Based on the causative agents, they are further classified into the following types:—

1.2.2.1.9.1 DEFICIENCY DISEASES

These diseases occur due to deficiency of some nutrients in the diet or deficient production of nutrients in the body. Some examples are night blindness due to deficiency of vitamin A, scurvy due to deficiency of vitamin C, rickets due to deficiency of vitamin D, goitre due to deficiency of iodine, dental caries due to deficiency of fluorine, etc. Other examples are diabetes mellitus due to deficiency of insulin and cretinism, myxoedema and goitre due to deficiency of thyroxine hormone, etc.

1.2.2.1.9.2 DEGENERATIVE DISEASES

These are organic diseases which occur due to degenerative changes in some vital organs of the body. Some examples are cardiovascular diseases (e.g. arteriosclerosis, atherosclerosis), cerebral strokes, epilepsy, osteoarthritis, rheumatoid arthritis, etc.

1.2.2.1.9.3 ALLERGIC DISEASES

These diseases are caused by certain substances (e.g. spores, pollens, certain foods) which on entering the human body produce allergic reactions. Some examples are hay fever, asthma, urticaria, etc. Certain human constitutions are hypersensitive to foreign substances called allergens.

1.2.2.1.9.4 CANCEROUS DISEASES

These diseases are caused by uncontrolled growth of cells in the body. The uncontrolled cell multiplications are triggered by some damaged proto-oncogenes or tumor-suppressor genes. The damages of such genes can be caused by carcinogenic substances like cigarette smoke, tobacco products, X-rays, nuclear radiations, ultraviolet rays, benzopyrene, automobile exhausts, etc. Majority of human cancers are found to be related to P 53 gene. Certain viruses (e.g. human papilloma virus) which are biological agents are also found to cause some cancers. Examples of these are cancers of uterine cervix. Cigarette smoke can cause lung cancer. Cadmium oxide can cause prostate cancer. Vinyl chloride can cause liver cancer.

1.3 OCCUPATIONAL DISEASES

These diseases develop in persons who are exposed to hazardous environment in their workplaces. For example, the persons who work with cutting, grinding and polishing of sandstones may suffer from a disease known as silicosis. The sand particles can cause irritation, inflammation and fibrosis of lung tissues. Similarly, an exposure to SO_2 from industries or air can cause irritation and suffocation in the human respiratory tract. A persistent exposure to it can also lead to asthma or bronchitis. NO_2 exposure can cause cancer. CO exposure can cause headache, dizziness, palpitation, suffocation and even death. Persistent exposure to metals in mines and smelter industries can cause respiratory tract diseases, heart diseases, CNS damage and cancer (e.g. from NI, CO)

1.4 AIDS AND HOMOEOPATHIC MEDICINES

This disease needs a special mention here because it is seriously affecting the humanity for last two decades as an incurable disease. It is a viral disease which overcomes the body's all defence mechanisms. It is caused by a retrovirus known as HIV (Human Immuno-deficiency Virus). More than 30 million people are now affected all over the world by HIV/AIDS infections. It is a disorder of cell-mediated immune system. HIV attacks helper T-lymphocytes. So, the number of T-cells drop, causing severe cellular immunodeficiency. The average incubation period is about 28 months. Only about 10% of the HIV infected persons develop full-blown AIDS. The rest act as carriers and spread the infections to others. Presently, tuberculosis is the main killer disease of HIV positive persons. The AIDS patients clinically develop some of the following symptoms:—

1. Lymphadenopathy (i.e. swelling of lymph nodes).

2. Lymphoma (i.e. cancer of lymphatics).

3. Thrombocytopenic purpurea (i.e. decreased blood platelets causing hemorrhage).

4. Kaposis sarcoma (a skin cancer).

5. Chronic encephalitis (i.e. severe brain damage).

6. A lung disease known as PCP (pneumocystis carinii pneumonia).

7. Wasting syndrome (i.e. substantial weight loss and decline in health).

8. AIDS-related complex (i.e. swollen lymph nodes, fever, night sweats, loss of weight, etc.).

If the AIDS symptoms are analysed clinically from the

homoeopathic point of view, there are homoeopathic remedies in the materia medica which have symptoms similar to the AIDS symptoms. These remedies can be efficacious in the treatment and management of AIDS. For example, for lymphadenopathy (i.e. swelling of lymph nodes), one of the most effective remedies is *Belladonna*. A few others are *Merc. sol.*, *Silicea* and *Tuberculinum* as intercurrents. For lymphoma (i.e. cancer of lymphatics), we can add to the list *Thuja, Hepar sulph., Calc. fluor., Arsenicum* in addition to the above set of remedies. For thrombocytopenic purpurea, there can be efficaceous remedies like *Phosphorus, Tuberculinum, Acid. nitricum* based on hemorrhagic tendency. For brain damage due to chronic encephalitis, *Psorinum* can be indicated based on the loss of memory, lack of ability to speak and inability to think.

In lung diseases known as PCP, *Tuberculinum* can be indicated. For wasting syndrome where there is substantial weight loss and decline in health, *Psorinum, Tuberculinum, Carbo veg., Iodium, Sulphur* may be indicated. For the symptoms of AIDS-related complex, *Tuberculinum* can be a well-indicated remedy. Kaposi's sarcoma, a skin cancer associated with AIDS clinically presents solitary or multiple, red brown, purple colored papules, nodules and plaques on the extremities (e.g. toes, legs below knee, fingers, face, scalp). Early lesions usually occur in toes or fingers. The lesions have a tendency to occur in clusters. They also occur bilaterally. Some lesions ulcerate. In children, there are striking, discrete, diffuse, nontender lymphadenopathy and hepatosplenomegaly. For lesions developing first at toes or lower legs and then spreading upward into fingers, face and scalp,

Ledum can be indicated. For lesions spreading from left to right *Lachesis*, from right to left *Lycopodium* and for ulcerating nodules *Hepar sulph.* may be indicated. For lymphadenopathy, *Belladonna* or *Tuberculinum* may be indicated. From the clinical symptoms picture, it is evident that AIDS shall be a multimiasmatic disease. All main miasms e.g. psoric, sycotic, syphilitic and tubercular shall play an important role in the evolution of a full-blown AIDS. So, intercurrent use of indicated miasmatic remedies (i.e. nosodes) shall be vital in successful management of AIDS.

1.5 REMARKS

Although therapeutic is the main objective of a clinician, it is necessary to know about a disease in all its aspects for its better management, treatment, prognosis and prevention. For example, in an infectious disease like chicken pox or small pox it is necessary to know about its cause, epidemiology, incubation period, symptoms, treatment and prophylaxis. In all these aspects, there exist information which can provide clues to homoeopathic remedy selection. For example, there is no modern vaccine against chicken pox. But chicken pox is caused by a virus known varicella. In homoeopathy, we have a remedy preparation known as *Varicillinum*. So, *Varicillinum* in 200th potency can be used as a prophylaxis for chicken pox to stimulate a short term, artificial immunity. It can also be used therapeutically. Some other prophylactic homoeopathic medicines are *Variolinum* for small pox, *Parotidinum* for mumps, *Diphtherinum* for diphtheria, *Morbillinum* for measles, *Psorinum* for tonsilitis, *Pertussin* for whooping cough, *Influenzinum* for viral fever, *Tuberculinum* for tuberculosis, asthmatic bronchitis, and pneumonia, etc. To develop a long-term immunity, it is necessary to use high potencies of the nosode remedies (i.e. vaccine equivalent medicines).

❖❖❖

CHAPTER-2

Background Methodologies In Homoeopathy

Master Hahnemann discovered homoeopathy in the year 1796. It was an unique event in the medical history of mankind. The fundamental law on which homoeopathy is based is known as the *'law of similars'*. According to this law, if the symptoms of a medicine and a disease are similar, then that medicine becomes curative for that disease. Now, the question arises what kinds of symptoms and what ways are to be considered to make and compare similarity between a disease and a remedy. There has been a lot of debate on this issue of symptom-similarity right from the days of master Hahnemann. This debate has led to innovations of a number of methodologies to search for simillimum (i.e. most similarity) by various masters of homoeopathy besides the classical method of Dr. Hahnemann. Some of the known methodologies are recapitulated here.

2.1 HAHNEMANNIAN TOTALITY

Dr. Hahnemann was very candid about the issue of symptom-similarity. In aphorism 6, he stated that a disease could be recognised and represented only by the *totality of its symptoms*. In aphorism 18, he further stressed that the totality of symptoms was the only indication and guide to the selection of an appropriate remedy for a disease. This is the classical concept of homoeopathy. When this concept of totality of symptoms is applied to a disease, the homoeopathic therapeutic becomes highly effective. In fact, every disease manifests a number of symptoms. In aphorism 152, Hahnemann states that the disease which has numerous striking symptoms shall certainly have a curative remedy. In aphorism 153, he further points out that in order to find the most suitable curative remedy, the totality of symptoms must include a few striking, singular, uncommon and peculiar (characteristic) symptoms. In aphorism 210, he also mentions that in all corporeal diseases the states of the patient's disposition (emotion) and mind are altered. So, he emphasized on the inclusion of the state of patient's disposition and mind in the ambit of totality of symptoms to evaluate the image of a disease more accurately.

In aphorism 5, 6 and 7, Hahnemann further calls for probing into the exciting or maintaining causes of a disease (causa occasionalis). He examplifies, in aphorism 173, some of the exciting causes which could be injurious to health. These are excessive food, insufficient food, less of sleep, physical chill, overheating of the body, dissipation of energy, physical strains, mental strains, physical irritation, excessive emotion, etc. For chronic diseases, Hahnemann, however, in aphorism 72, states that the chronic diseases are caused by dynamic infections with chronic miasms (e.g. psora, sycosis, syphilis). In aphorism 6, he points out that all perceptible signs and symptoms put together shall only represent the disease phenomenon in its entireity. And it shall be the true picture of a totality of symptoms. The signs and symptoms are collected mainly from three kinds of sources. On these, Hahnemann in aphorism 6, states that the changes in the health of a body and mind are perceived by the patient through sensations, remarked by those around the patient, and observed by the physician himself.

It is true that Hahnemannian method of totality is a cumbersome procedure but it is an infallible method of treatment. It is true that it is often difficult to retrieve the Hahnemannian totality at a first interview. It is more often so for most of the beginners who enter directly in the field of clinical practices after formal education without former experience.

2.2 KENT'S CONSTITUTION

Homoeopathy did not halt at the concept of totality of symptoms as enunciated in aphorism 6. After Hahnemann, several masters of homoeopathy attempted finding simillimum in more and more number of ways. Prominent among them were Dr. Boenninghausen, Dr. Hering, Dr. Kent and some others, and more recently Dr. George Vithoulkas, Dr. Jan Scholten, Dr. Rajan Sankaran and a few others. They built up further on the foundation of the law of similars. It helped to grow and develop homoeopathy into some more new areas. It is a fact that similarities can exist at different levels of the diseases, human bodies and remedies. They also exist in various forms, ways and degrees. It is the quality, quantity and content of similarities which are considered by various physicians to put forward their concepts of similarities. All the later suggested methods are innovative in their own ways and are found equally effective in the treatment of various human diseases.

Kent's concept of constitutional remedies is an excellent addition to the system of homoeopathy. When similarities are observed between the various constitutional levels of a sick person and a remedy, the remedy cures the disease. Kent's method of going generals to particulars provided enough signs and symptoms to determine a constitutional remedy. The constitutional remedy seems to rectify one's constitutional imbalances and susceptibilities, inherited or acquired. I cite here in brief the characteristics of a few well-known constitutional remedies. For example, *Calcarea carbonica* has a constitution which is fat, fair, flabby, cold, pale, moist, slow, sluggish, compassionate, delicate, polished, shy, timid, sensitive, mild, soft, indecisive, lacking self-confidence, perspiring locally, prone to anxiety and fear, susceptible to cold. It gets easily tired and exhausted, both physically and mentally. It desires egg, sweet, sour, salt, meat, butter, lime, chalk, tea, vinegar or some stimulants. It has a fear of darkness and disease, particularly heart disease and cancer. It is aggravated from cold air, cold water, overexertion, hurry, worry and tension.

On the other hand, *Arsenicum album* has a constitution which is restless, irritable, chilly, sensitive, neat, tidy, fastidious, nervous, highly strung, selfish, not-too-ambitious, not interested to take much responsibility, artistic in work, always feel insecured, has aristocratic look with thin hands and face, perspires easily and profusely, likes accuracy and details, allergic to cold and slight change of temperature, possesses much anxiety about health, has fear of disease particulary of cancer, always needs support from the people around, desires company, takes frequent sips of water. It is aggravated from slightest cold, cold water, cold air, 1-2 A.M., 1-2 P.M., physical exertion. It has a fear that he will die if left alone.

Nux vomica has a constitution which is usually male, intelligent, highly irritable, bad tempered, hyperactive, chilly, easily offended, overworked, mentally strained, highly efficient, a great goal setter and achiever, works upto late hours of night, desires stimulant , alcohol, cigarette, coffee, has high-flying life style, constipation, dyspepsia, headache, piles, sleeplessness, demands high degree of efficiency from others, prone to violence, anger and short temper. *Sulphur,* a chronic of *Nux vomica,* is another great constitutional remedy. It is stoop-shouldered, warm blooded, quick tempered, touchy, easily offended, selfish, egoist, proudy, independent, untidy in appearance, dress and habit, ragged philosopher, averse to be washed, has dry, rough and unhealthy skin, sweats profusely, offensive body odor, redness of all orifices, susceptible to skin diseases, burning of soles, epigastric discomfort, likes sweets, salts and meat. It is aggravated at 12 noon and 12 night.

2.3 BOENNINGHAUSEN'S GRAND SYMPTOM

Dr. Von Boenninghausen put forword a concept of searching similarity through four different spheres of a disease. These were designated as location, sensation, modality and concomitant. In his view, these four categories of symptoms put together known as Grand symptom have enough basis to indicate a simillimum. In fact, this methodology often provided a quick and effective way of remedy selection. By location it is meant the site of localisation of a disease or the chief complaint. For example, a migraine (headache) may be located on the right side or left side or vertex or occipital region of the head. Similarly, a pain may be localised in the liver or spleen or epigastrium or heart or kidney or gall bladder or ureter or right chest or left chest, etc. There can be many such examples. Some remedies have location affinities as found in their provings. For example, *Lycopodium* has effect on the right side or R —>L side, and *Lachesis* on the left side or L —> R side, and *Lac caninum* on alternate sides of human body. Some remedies have also organ specificities. For example, *Chelidonium* for liver, *Ceanothus americanus* for spleen, *Carduus marianus* for gall bladder, *Berberis vulgaris* for kidney, *Crataegus oxycantha* for heart, etc.

By sensation of the grand symptom, it is meant to be a perceived sensation or a feeling of the affected person during his sickness. It may be a locally perceived sensation, or a generalised sensation of the whole body. For example, a pain felt in the appendicular area during an acute attack of appendicitis may be a stitching pain (like *Bryonia, Kali. carb.*), or a contracting pain (like *Colocynth, Causticum, Rhus tox.*). Similarly, a patient may feel chilly (like *Nux vomica*) or warm sensation (like *Bryonia*) during an acute attack of appendicitis. A woman at menopause often feels alternate cold and hot flushes in her body (like *Pulsatilla, Tuberculinum*). During an acute attack of a malarial fever, a patient may feel chill and rigor periodically (like *Arsenicum album, China, Nutrium muriaticum*). A person may also feel cold or hot bodily because of his constitutional endowment. That is why some persons dislike cold climate because of having cold-blooded constitutions (e.g. *Arsenicum album, Nux vomica, Calcarea carbonica*). Similarly, some persons dislike hot climate because of having warm-blooded constitutions (e.g. *Pulsatilla, Lycopodium, Sulphur*). Also, some persons are sensitive to both cold and hot climates (e.g. *Merc. sol.*).

Modality is another important sphere of symptom collection and evaluation. It is an aggravated or ameliorated state of a symptom under certain influencing conditions. For example, a *Bryonia* state is aggravated from the slightest of movement and relieved while at rest. Opposite is the *Rhus tox.* state which is aggravated from a restful condition and relieved by movements. There are also time modalities. For example, *a Lycopodium* state can be aggravated between 4 PM to 8 PM, *Arsenicum album* state between 1 AM to 2 AM or 1 PM to 2 PM, *Kali. bichrome* state between 2 AM to 3 AM, *Kali. carb.* state from 2 AM to 5 AM, *Sulphur* state at 12 noon or 12 night, etc. Climatic conditions also affect the degree of symptom development. For example, a *Rhus tox.* state of asthma or gouty pain is aggravated during the rainy season or a bad weather or a cloudy weather. Even, the lunar variations can influence the symptom state. For example, a Silicea state of asthma or arthritic pain is aggravated during full Moon and new Moon.

Concomitants are another set of valuable symptoms for remedy selection. They may or may not be directly related to the chief complaint or principal disease. There may be a feeling of nausea (e.g. *Ipecac*) or a state of convulsion (e.g. *Balladonna, Cuprum met.*) concomitant to a fever. There may be a lot of salivation from the mouth (e.g. *Merc. sol.*) during a fever. There may be a thick, milky, white-coat on the surface of tongue (e.g. *Antim. crude*) during a fever or a diarrhea. There can also be manifestation of some mental symptoms concomitant to physical ailments. For example, there may be a fear of death (e.g. *Aconite*) or anxiety and restlessness (e.g. *Arsenicum album*), or mental depression (e.g. *Ignatia*), or anger and irritability (e.g. *Hepar sulph., Nux vomica, Chamomilla*) during a fever. Sometimes, there may be expression of some peculiar concomitant symptoms. For example, there may be much thirsty feeling for cold water during the chilly phase of a fever (e.g. *Natrium muriaticum*). Similarly, there can be complete thirstlessness for water during a high fever inspite of dryness of mouth, tongue and throat (e.g. *Pulsatilla*). Boenninghausen's grand symptom is in fact an easily and quickly comprehensible method to search for simillimum in many cases.

2.4 HERING'S LAW OF CURE

It is an outstanding law proposed by Dr. Constantine Hering to verify the action mechanism of a medicine. This verification is necessary to confirm whether a medicine is working in the right direction or not. A physician should be in a position to rightly follow the curative process of an administered drug. Hering's law states that:—

(a) A right cure proceeds in the human body from above downward.

(b) A right cure moves in the human body from within outward.

(c) A right cure starts from the most important organ and proceeds to the least important organ of the human body.

(d) A right cure moves in the reverse order of appearance of symptoms in the human body.

Any one or more of the above four vectoral phenomena can be observed if the interaction between a disease and a medicine is closely followed. If these rules are not followed in a curative process, a radical cure cannot be expected. It can be explained by a simple phenomenon. For example, in a diabetic patient, the blood sugar, whether fasting or post-prandial, is the ultimate pathological manifestation. While treating a diabetic patient, the blood sugar level has to show some reduction at first instance in the curative process after the administration of a simillimum medicine. So, a frequent monitoring of blood sugar level is to be done at appropriate intervals. If higher blood sugar level is not reduced after an optimum waiting period, the medicine is not working for the diabetic patient. The pancreatic disorder which is the source cannot be cured unless the higher level of blood sugar which is the end product cannot be reduced or controlled.

Let us now take an example of a viral disease (e.g. measles). It is known that measles eruptions start from the mouth and face and then spread downward from the upper part to the lower part of the body. After administration of a homoeopathic remedy, the measles eruptions should disappear in the reverse order of their appearance. A true curative process shall start form the lower part of the body (e.g. legs) and gradually shall move upward into the upper part of the body (e.g. hands, face). This phenomenon can easily be observed by a beginner as a test case of study.

As clinical observations expand, Hering's law helps us to further extend the principle and apply it in different spheres of human body. For example, the highermost organ of human body is brain. Sometimes, we come across brain tumors (e.g. pituitary tumors) in young girls having long standing amenorrhea. It is a sure sign of regression of tumors if the menses are re-established in those girls after administration of simillimum remedies. The pituitary tumors can sometimes cause blurring of vision or blindness to patients. If after the administration of simillimum remedies, blindness or blurred vision are improved, it is the indication of regression of the brain tumors. The eye symptoms are improved as the tumors diminish in size if the Hering's law is applied.

Again, mental symptoms are the products of functions of human brain. So, they (i.e. mental symptoms) are given highest values in remedy evaluation. In a curative process, thus, the mental symptoms should be relieved first prior to the physical symptoms. For example, a patient may come with a hypertension which has developed in him after a strong fearful incident. After the administration of *Aconite* in high potency, his fear of mind disappears first and then slowly his hypertension is reduced. Since here, both mental and physical spheres of symptom are involved in the sickness, the curative process starts from the mental sphere although the physical symptom (e.g. hypertension) has developed later. In this case, Hering's law does not follow the reverse order of chronological appearance. But in the case of diabetes mellitus the rule follows the reverse order of appearance of symptoms because, there, both the symptoms (e.g. the disorder in pancreatic cells and the higher sugar level in blood) belong to the physical sphere of human being. If mental and physical spheres are both involved in a sickness, the right cure moves from the mental sphere to the physical sphere.

2.5 GEORGE VITHOULKAS' ESSENCES

In recent times, Dr.George Vithoulkas' work had been an outstanding contribution to the field of homoeopathy. He put forward a novel concept of essence remedies. According to him, the homoeopathic remedies can be explained in terms of mental-emotional essences as their central themes. For example, he considers *Bryonia* to be endowed with a central theme of loneliness and insecurity. They (*Bryonia*) are withdrawn and isolated from social contacts. They feel anger, irritability and resentment when disturbed, physically or mentally. An image of *Bryonia* can be built up on these themes. Similarly, in *Hepar sulph.*, the central themes are oversensitivity and abusiveness. Their nerves are always on the edges. They are prone to violence, anger, irritability, contempt, verbal abuse and intolerance. On the other hand, the essence of *Acid. nitricum* is dissatisfaction.

They are always dissatisfied. They have great dissatisfaction about health, treatment and physician. But they are not abusive like *Hepar sulph.*

According to Vithoulkas, *Arsenicum album* has an essence that is constituted of deep-seated insecurity, dependency, selfishness, possessiveness and fastidiousness. They always feel vulnerable, defenceless and insecured about their health. So, they become restless, anxious, fastidious, tidy, neat and clean. They have a deep fear of death. So, they seek constant support and company from others. They fear loneliness. On the other hand, *Nux vomica* has an essence of ambition, competitiveness, achievement. They are self-reliant, hard working, impulsive, fastidious about efficiency. They have strong sense of duty and work ethics. They crave stimulants.

In *Phosphorus,* the essence of the remedy is diffusion. There is diffusion at mental, emotional and physical level. Because of emotional diffusion, they are frank, warm, friendly, extrovert, outgoing, affectionate and sympathetic. They can express themselves effortlessly. Diffusion at physical level make them vulnerable to bleed easily from any organ or parts of the body. There can be nose bleeding, hemoptysis, hemorrhoids, hematuria or uterine hemorrhage in *Phosphorus* patients. In *Aurum metallicum,* the essence is mental depression and loathing of life. They are honest, just, fair, serious and responsible people. So, they are vulnerable to any dent in interpersonal relationships. They are closed people. They do not express their feelings easily. As a result, they suffer internally and move towards mental depression. They are touchy and sensitive to criticisms. In this way, all remedies of the materia medica can be explained with the help of their individual essences.

2.6 JAN SCHOLTEN'S GROUP ANALYSIS

It is another innovative way of searching simillimum from the kingdom of minerals and chemical elements. In his work, Dr. Jan Scholten describes the characteristic themes of a group of chemical elements or cations or anions of a mineral and then combines the central themes of the composing elements to deduce the total symptom picture of a remedy. For example, he brings out the group symptoms of cations like *Calcium, Magnesium, Potassium, Sodium (Natrium)*, and anions like chloride (*Muriaticum*), carbonate (*Carbonicum*), sulphate (*Sulphuricum*), nitrate (*Nitricum*), fluoride (*Floratum*), iodide (*Iodatum*), etc. To understand the image of *Calcarea carbonica,* he considers seperately the group symptoms of calcium and carbonicum (i.e. carbonate) as follows :

Calcium

What do others think

Sensitive to critisism

Insensitivity

Shyness

Fears

Protection

Withdrawal

Carbonicum

Giving meaning

Stating values

Self worth

Dignity

Shyness

Worker

Father

When combined together, the ideas constitute a total picture of *Calcarea carbonica*. If it is desired to know *Kali. carb.* picture, then the themes of kalium (i.e. potassium) is added to the themes of carbonicum. The Kalium is considered to have the following themes:—

Principle or duty
Closed
Optimism
Work, task
Family

Similarly, for *Natrium mur.,* the themes of Natrium (i.e. sodium) and muriaticum (i.e. chloride) are considered together. Seperately, they have the following group symptoms:—

Natrium	**Muriaticum**
Sadness	Self pity
Depression	Care
Closed, alone	Nurturing
Restriction	Mother
Denial, forbidden	Attention
Sensitive	Self awareness
Holding on	

While considered singly, the element remedy *Phosphorus* (i.e. phosphoricum) has the following themes:—

Communication
Sympathetic
Friends, acquaintances, neighbors
Brothers
Homesickness
Curiosity and travel
Restlessness and fears

The above examples have been cited only to demonstrate how a remedy picture can be understood by using the group analysis of Dr. Jan Scholten. For details, his two books are important referrals.

2.7 RAJAN SANKARAN'S METHODS OF DELUSION, CENTRAL DISTURBANCE AND SITUATIONAL MATERIA MEDICA

According to Dr. Sankaran (1997), a delusion can be considered as a false perception of a situation of realities. He considers delusion to be a much underused rubric of the repertory. A delusion can play a greater role in the selection of simillimum. In delusions, there are also exaggerated levels of normal feelings. For example, one delusion of *Thuja* is " as if he is made of glass". According to Sankaran, this delusion means that the person has a feeling of being very delicate, brittle and fragile. He feels that this state can lead to a break up of his body. This is an exaggerated feeling of fragility expressed by *Thuja* patients. Sankaran further adds that the delusion has another important component known as fixity of ideas (i.e. fixed ideas). The delusion can also lead to other feelings and expressions which are linked to, or are consequences of it. Many remedies can be selected on the basis of their delusions, or the delusions can be used to differentiate remedies.

Dr. Sankaran put forward another innovative concept of Central disturbance. According to him, a disease is not something local but a disturbance of the whole being. If the disturbance at the centre is treated, the local problems are also lessened. He states that the central disturbance being same all over, the easy way to identify it is to understand the mental state of a patient. He gives an example with *Kali. iod.*, which he identifies in a patient of leucoderma. The patient was very expressive, humorous and jocular during interview in spite of having a total skin discoloration. A state of mind such as " loquacity with jesting" was considered to represent the central disturbance which led to *Kali. iod.* According to Sankaran, modalities can also represent central disturbances in some cases. He gives an example with *Bryonia*, which has aggravation from the least motion. In a *Bryonia* patient, even a little movement of finger may worsen a pain in the knee. Such is the degree of acuteness of his central disturbance.

Another novel idea of Dr. Sankaran is *'Situational Materia Medica'*. He considers it to be an original situation from which the present state of a remedy has been derived. He gives an example with *Calcarea silicata,* which has an anxiety about money matters and a fear of poverty. This mental state of *Calcarea silicata* develops due to a situation that he comes from a family background of poor financial status. So, a *Calcarea silicata* patient is very careful about spending. He is yielding type, he cannot assert himself, he has lack of self-confidence, he depends on people socially and financially, he behaves like a pauper, he is sensitive to reprimand, he is timid, he is fearful. All these characteristics of *Calcarea silicata* are considered to have come from his original situation of poverty which Sankaran calls a *"Situational Materia Medica"*.

On the other hand, a Silicate state is considered to have come from a rich or sound financial background. So, a *Silicea* patient behaves like a prince. He is obstinate, he is rigid, he is conscientious, he tries to reach high ideals. In this way, by using the original situations, the subsequent evolution of mental states can be understood for many remedies of the materia medica.

2.8 THEMATIC DETERMINATION OF CANCER REMEDIES

Recently, the author (Roy, 2000), put forward a concept of identifying cancer-susceptible remedies in his book *"Homoeopathy in cancer treatment"*. This methodology is based on a fundamental principle that is convertibility of physical symptoms into mental symptoms (states) and vice-versa. The thematic principle was derived from the observations that the symptom development seemed to be always a two-way phenomenon. Whenever there is a disturbance at the physical level, there is a concomitant disturbance at the mental level and vice-versa. A very subtle change in the mental state may not be always appropriated by a patient who is not acutely sensitive. But it (i.e. any minute change of mental state) shall always remain at his subconscious level. For example, a state of breathlessness in a patient can cause an anxiety in him. Similarly, a state of anxiety in the subject can also cause a breathlessness in him. Only the forms and intensity of two symptoms which are interchangeable and intercommunicable between the body and mind are different. One is called clinical disease (e.g. breathlessness) while the other is called mental state (e.g. anxiety). So, clinical disease and mental state seem to be interrelated, interdependent and interchangeable phenomena. In other words, it can be said that physical and mental symptoms are transformable to one another like conversion of one form of energy into another. This phenomenon can be represented by a reversible symbol as follows:—

Physical symptoms $\rightleftarrows$ Mental symptoms(states)

Now using this thematic principle, various cancer-susceptible remedies and their sensitivity to different clinical stages of malignancy can be worked out. The clinical characteristics of malignant tumors and dynamic behaviors of malignant cells can be transformed into repertorial rubrics of mind. It seems plausible because there is a kind of pattern in the behavior of malignant cells and their growths. The phenomenon of mutual conversion of physical and mental symptoms into one another can be well recognised. An example of using the thematic principle is that an advanced malignant tumor is usually very hard and rigid by nature in the physical sense. Such tumor is also very resistant to treatment and difficult to be therapeutically resolved. These physical characteristics of an advanced stage malignant tumor can be thematically transformed into appropriate repertorial rubrics of mind e.g. obstinate, disobedience, defiant, etc. The rubrics: obstinancy, disobediance and defiance are some of the characteristics of the nosode remedy *Tuberculinum*. So, according to this thematic principle, *Tuberculinum* can be an effective remedy in the treatment of advanced cancer.

Similarly, in the early stage of malignancy, cancer is almost asymptomatic. It eludes early detection. From its pre-cancer stage, the disease progressess silently to the state of malignancy. In early stage, a fundamental character of malignancy is its hiding tendency (rubric: desire to hide). In this sense, the disease has a tendency to deceive its own host (rubrics: deceiptful, sly, dishonest). Also, pre-cancer lesions like leukoplakia, erythroplakia, giant pigmented moles, genital warts, dysplasia, etc., are all ugly looking in the physical sense. So, in pre-cancers and early cancers, we get a theme of ugliness, hiding tendency, deceiptfulness, slyness, secretiveness. All these characteristics are observed in the sycotic remedy *Thuja occidentalis*. So, *Thuja* can be an effective remedy in differnt types of pre-cancer and early cancer.

In this way, by using the thematic principle, most of the remedies of materia medica can be analysed for their cancer-susceptibility and their degree of sensitivity (i.e. efficacy) to various clinical stages. From the use of the thematic principle of convertibility of symptoms, it is found that many of the potential remedies of materia medica still remain unused, underused or neglected for cancer therapy. Some of the prominent underused remedies are *Belladonna, Tarentula, Tuberculinum, Hyoscyamus, Stramonium*, etc. These remedies have their cancer-susceptibilities (i.e. inherent efficacy), although the final selection of a remedy in a particular case shall depend upon the individual Hahnemannian peculiarity.

For early cancer remedies, we can use the following rubrics:—

Hide, desire to (SR-575)

Deceiptful, sly (SR-201)

Dishonest (SR-412)

Mischievous (SR-743)

For advanced cancer remedies, we can use the following rubrics:—

Defiant (SR-202)

Disobedience (SR-413)

Obstinate (SR-787)

Violent, vehement (SR-1055)

Destructiveness (SR-397)

Rage, fury(SR-813)

Cruelty, inhumanity(SR-190)

Unfeeling, hard hearted (SR-1053)

Hatred (SR-570)

Malicious, spiteful, vindictive(SR-720)

Wander, desire to (SR-1061)

Travel, desire to (SR-1030)

For terminal cancer remedies, we can use the following rubrics:—

Kill, desire to (SR-682)

Threatening(SR-1020)

Kill, threatens to (SR-1021)

Destroy, threatens to (SR-1020)

Threatens destruction and death (SR-64)

Using the above rubrics, *Hepar sulph., Silicea, Tarentula, Tuberculinum, Nux vomica, Hyoscyamus, Stramonium, Merc. sol., Syphilinum, Lach., Lyc., Arsenicum, Belladonna, Anacardium, Alumina, Agaricus,* etc. are found to have basic susceptibility to terminal cancers. The thematic principle holds potential to be utilised in cases of other diseases also, where there is a kind of conspicuously identifiable pattern in their clinical behavior. I cite here an example. Recently, I used this thematic principle for determination of a similar remedy in a case of a severe rheumatoid arthritis of wrist joints in a middle aged woman. She had been suffering from the disease for last five years for which she was on allopathic medication. She was on steroids and analgesic tablets. She got acute pain, stiffness, rigidity and swelling of the wrist joints < movement, exertion, rest, morning. All indicated remedies like *Bryonia, Rhus tox., Medorrhinum* failed to relieve her on long term. Then, by converting the themes of physical rigidity, hardness, stiffness, lack of flexibility of the joints, nagging pain, and closing of the joints space into appropriate repertorial rubrics of mind (e.g. obstinancy, rigidity of mind, fixed ideas, irritability, closed, sclerosed, inflexibility of mind), *Kali. carb.* was selected and it was given in 200C/2D/ 12 hourly. The remedy brought in spectacular relief of the entire condition of wrist joints. The pain, swelling and rigidity gradually subsided. The relief continued to persist for long. So, the thematic principle needs to be applied and verified in more and more cases where there are paucity of characteristic symptoms (i.e. one-sided diseases of master, Hahnemann) and incurable chronic diseases (e.g. Alzheimer's, Parkinson's, multiple sclerosis, cancer, AIDS, etc.).

2.9 RECOGNITION OF CERTAIN PROBLEMS

Master Hahnemann considered the entire aspect of a disease to collect its totality of symptoms. A disease may have a number of symptoms, subjective and objective. The subject shall have his own constitutional symptoms. He shall also have his miasmatic characteristics (e.g. psoric, sycotic, syphilitic, tubercular). There can be some causative and influencing factors as well for a disease. There can be concomitant mental and emotional dispositions of a subject. There can also be other concomitants, particulars and peculiars. There can be local symptoms and general symptoms. When symptoms from all these spheres are collected and considered together, the simillimum becomes infallible. This is the true Hahnemannian way of collecting totality of symptoms. Therefore, Hahnemann, in aphorism 18, states that totality of symptoms is the only guide to and indication for a simillimum remedy. It is the classical concept of remedy selection. However, it is not always easy to reach Hahnemannian simillimum during a bed-side prescription. Many of the beginners complain of not being able to practice Hahnemannian simillimum. It is like not reaching an actual homoeopathic fulfilment. Some may grow with disillusionment, some with discontentment, some with lack of confidence, some with disappointment and some with polypharmacy. Some may end up even leaving Homoeopathy, an outstanding healing technique and a noble profession, to take up some unrelated careers. It is the collective responsibility of all pre-eminent homoeopaths to prevent such drift of neophytes from the field of homoeopathy and stop this predicament. This can ensure a better survival and further progress of homoeopathic therapeutics.

It is first and foremost requirement of every student of homoeopathy to nurture Hahnemannian concept of totality to be a more successful practitioner. Other methods need to be learnt and utilised wherever and whenever applicable. But Hahnemannian similarity is universally applicable to all cases of ailments if it can be worked out. It is true that working out a Hahnemannian simillimum is an arduous, difficult and cumbersome task. It is not the concept alone which matters. It is also the way we approach it, analyse it, understand it, comprehend it and apply it often what matters for the beginners. It is in this context that a different approach was formulated in this book to explain in an easily comprehensible way the Hahnemannian totality of symptoms and its further spin-offs. The discussed concept of approach was derived not on the basis of any theoretical consideration but it was indicated from observations of numerous clinical situations and results of their treatments. Practically, the concept is found to be applicable in each and every case of diseases and health disorders of human beings.

❖❖❖

CHAPTER-3

Conceptualisation

3.1 THE CONCEPT EVOLUTION

Over the years after dealing with a large number of human diseases, I could observe some new ways of analysing, understanding, considering and explaining the Hahnemannian totality. These observations led to the conceptualisation of a systematised, comprehensive and effective way of dealing with diseases, their treatment and management. The basic concept that emerged from such observations is that every human sickness (i.e. disease/disorder) consisted of three essential components. These can be termed as:—

(i) Cause of the disease,

(ii) Manifestation of the actual disease, and

(iii) Effect of the disease.

All diseases, acute or chronic, shall be made up of these three component elements which together, in essence, represent the

Hahnemannian totality. Schematically, the entity of a human sickness, small or big, can be split into the following components:—

Human sickness ⎡ Cause
⎢ Disease(sensustricto)
⎣ Effect

3.2 CAUSE

Any disease can be explained in terms of the above three constituent phenomena i.e. *causative phenomenon, disease phenomenon and effect phenomenon.* For example, a patient may come with a fever to a physician. He may tell that he contracted this fever after going out into the scorching heat of the Sun (e.g. *Gelsemium*), or after getting drenched in rains (e.g. *Dulcamara*), or after a fearful incident (e.g. *Aconite*). Similarly, a patient may come with an abdominal pain. He may tell that he got this pain after eating some meat (e.g. *Pulsatilla*), or after some worm infestations (e.g. *Cina*), or after an emotional upset (e.g. *Ignatia*). In all these cases, the causative backgrounds of the ailments are clearly known. Hence, the causative phenomena guide to the simillimum remedies. But even after deposition by the patients, a physician must verify through enquiries the accuracy of their statements and the true nature of the causative events. In the *Organon of Medicine,* master Hahnemann himself emphasized on these causative aspects of diseases. I prefer to call them as causative phenomena (C) because they involve a series of interactions before influencing the patients. In aphorism 5, Hahnemann directs us to discover the most probable exciting cause of an acute disease and fundamental cause in the whole history of a chronic disease. He called the maintaining cause of a disease as *"causa occasionalis"*. Similarly, he considered chronic miasm to be one of the fundamental causes of chronic diseases. The human constitutions and miasms can be considered to belong to causative phenomena because, in many cases, miasmatic and constitutional susceptibilities predispose individual subjects to contract, maintain and recur diseases. For example, *Arsenicum, Phosphorus, Calcarea carb., Graphites* and *Sepia* constitutions are susceptible to develop cancer. *Bryonia, Rhus tox.* and *Kali. carb* constitutions are likely to develop arthritis, rheumatism, spondylitis (cervical and lumbar), etc.

3.2 DISEASE

Where the exact cause of the disease is not identifiable because either the patient could not perceive it well or he could no remember it, it is necessary to look for disease symptoms or the effect symptoms to work out a simillimum. In aphorism 7, Hahnemann says that in a disease where there is no manifested exciting or maintaining cause we must regard the morbid symptoms which shall point to a suitable remedy. I prefer to call these morbid symptoms as disease phenomenon (D). Broadly, it covers all the symptoms of an actual disease represented by location, sensation, modality and concomitant of Boenninghausen. All these symptoms can constitute a disease phenomenon. The characteristic symptoms, if available, in the disease sphere may also indicate a simillimum. Let us now consider an example of an acute case. Say, a patient comes with a fever for which he does not remember any causative situation which might have triggered the disease. But he can describe the disease symptoms well. He says that he feels very thirsty during the fever, he has constipated stool, he gets much relief from taking rest, he has a concomitant frontal headache, he gets irritated and disturbed by any kind of noise, movement, light or phone call. So, here, the disease symptoms clearly guide to a simillimum remedy which is likely to be *Bryonia*. In this case, although the cause of the disease is not known, we can still select the simillimum based on symptoms of the disease phenomenon.

Now, let us consider a chronic case where both the causative factor and the disease phenomenon can be combined together to select a simillimum. Say, a patient comes with a long-standing pain of his right arm, from shoulder to fingers. Pain is accompanied with a feeling of numbness. His complaint is aggravated by keeping the arm hanging down. A peculiar concomitant is excessive gas formation and fullness of abdomen. He feels thirsty at night. He has constipated stool. Constitutionally, he is short, thin and rigid, very quick, intelligent, analytical, domineering, warm blooded, susceptible to chronic dysentery, has desire for sweets. He is forgetful. He feels nervousness before an ordeal. Here, the causative phenomenon is his constitutional susceptibility. His disease symptoms and constitutional characteristics together indicate *Lycopodium* to be his simillimum remedy.

3.4 EFFECT

A third great element of similarity which is clearly identifiable in the whole milieu of a human sickness can be termed as *'effect of the disease'*. I prefer to call it an effect phenomenon (E). Every disease shall have an effect, small or big, mildly or strongly perceptible, prominent or not prominent, transient or permanent. The effect phenomenon can be visible or perceptible on physical, mental and emotional levels. It shall also be expressed by signs and symptoms, visible to the physician, or perceived by the patient, or expressed by the persons around the patient. The effect phenomenon either in combination with other phenomena or independently if characteristics can indicate a simillimum. Many a times, it happens that the cause-based remedy or the symptom from the disease sphere are not able to indicate the simillimum, or they fail to effect a permanent cure. In such cases, the effect phenomenon if pronounced can indicate a simillimum. The absence of any characteristic symptom from the causative or disease sphere is not any contraindication. If symptoms from the effect sphere are sufficiently pronounced, they can act as an indicator for a simillimum. I cite here below a small case example:—

A lady aged 35 years came with a complaint of frequent menses for last three years. She had taken a lot of treatment from gynecological specialists with no permanent solution. An USG scan showed no abnormalities in the uterus. Because of her long-standing suffering, using many types of medicines, and hearing all kinds of frightening words from neighbors and friends she had been worrying a lot. Long drawn and persistent worrying has led her to a state of mind which is now charactarised by dullness, gloom, sadness, hopelessness, listlessness, introversion, loneliness, sobbing and sighing. This state of mind is not her original disease but it has developed due to her long-lasting suffering from the principal physical disease (i.e. frequent menstrual bleeding for three years) and constant worrying because of it. Her present mental state can be called what is an effect of the principal disease, or simply an effect phenomenon.

Since sufficiently characteristic symptoms were not available from the causative sphere or the disease sphere, she was given *Ignatia* 200C/3D/12 hourly based on the effect symptoms. The remedy brought in a spectacular recovery of her mental state and the physical disease stopping the frequent bleeding and regularising the menses. The recovery brought a great deal of relief to the patient and her family.

In another case, a middle aged man, 36 years in age, came with a diabetic complaint which was there for last six months. He was on allopathic Daonil tablet. His latest blood sugar was F=168 mg/dl and PP=265 mg/dl. His disease (i.e. diabetes) symptoms were not much characteristic. His thirst for water was normal. Appetite was good. He liked normal sour, salt and chilies. There was no special desire/aversion. Urine was not very frequent. He lost his body weight from 84 Kg to 66 Kg. But his main bodily complaint was a feeling of a strong neck pain which extended to his occipital region. He told whenever his blood sugar was higher, the neck pain increased. There was also stiffness in the neck and he got relief by neck exercises. He was a chilly patient. On his prominent neck symptoms which were probably the consequences (e.g. neuropathic) of his diabetes. He was given *Rhus tox.* 200C/3 doses/12 hourly. The remedy gave him a great relief of his neck pain and stiffness and also reduced his blood sugar level. After one month, his blood sugar was F=130 mg/dl. and PP=185 mg/dl. Since the disease symptoms and constitutional symptoms were not very characteristic, his remedy was selected based on some prominent effect symptoms of the disease. At that point of time, the effect symptoms which were strongly marked guided to the simillimum. Under normal rule of homoeopathic practice, those neck symptoms shall be designated as *'concomitant symptoms'*. But in reality, those neck symptoms were neuropathic consequences of his diabetic condition. So, effect symptoms can guide to the simillimum where disease symptoms and causative symptoms are not pronounced.

The effect phenomenon can also be understood from the following example. For instance, a patient comes with a chronic throat trouble (e.g. chronic pharyngitis). He may tell that he had been taking various treatments for long without any permanent relief. He gets throat irritation, pain and coughing from time to time, get < cold weather. He has a sensation as if there is something stuck up in the throat. He has developed an inner anxiety about the disease. He is apprehensive that he may develop some serious disease. He worries constantly about his throat trouble. He fears that the throat trouble may ultimately turn out to be a cancer. So, he is anxious, worried, afraid and restless. He moves from doctor to doctor. This mental state is exactly what is meant to be the effect phenomenon of his disease. In this case, *Acid. nitricum* is likely to be the simillimum. Similarly, a disorder in the mental state of a subject can also lead to some physical disorders and vice-versa. So, an outstanding effect phenomenon if available can be used as an essence to indicate a simillimum.

3.5 TWO TYPES OF MENTALS

Such effect phenomenon(E) can be observed in many cases and are usually termed as mental symptoms as a general rule. It is certainly a group of mental symptoms. But this phenomenon of mental symptoms needs to be differentiated from other kinds of mental symptoms. The mental symptoms can be classified into two basic types. There are also fundamental differences between these two types. One group of mental symptoms arise due to the effect of a disease while the other group of mental symptoms occur as natural endowment of a constitutional entity. The first group can be called '*effect phenomenon*' while the second category can be called '*constitutional characteristics*'.

3.6 THREE DYNAMIC PHENOMENA

The cause, disease and effect of a human sickness have been suffixed by the word '*phenomenon*' because they represent some changes from the normal state of human health and mind. Hence, the terminologies are used as '*causative phenomenon*', '*disease phenomenon*' and '*effect phenomenon*'. They can be either combined into a group of two or three phenomena, or considered singly if pronounced and characteristic to indicate simillimum. If history and symptoms of a disease are taken meticulously, all three phenomena can be observed, distinguished and separated unambiguously in a given case of a sickness and utilised as essences to work out the most suitable remedy. Every disease if analysed and understood in terms of the above three spheres of symptoms development, it becomes easier to comprehend the Hahnemannian similarity (i.e. totality) which leads to greater successes in homoeopathic remedy applications.

3.7 SYNTHESIS

Each and every case of a sickness shall consist of three distinct components e.g. cause, disease/disorder and effect. This is a universal law of the Nature. It is a different matter whether all three components of a sickness can be delineated or not in every case. But their existence is unequivocal. Even, the infectious diseases have causative factors like bacteria or virus or fungus. But, in such cases, the homoeopathic remedy selection depends upon the disease phenomenon or effect phenomenon because these remedies have not been proved based on their disease-causing organisms. For example, in infectious diseases like typhoid, tuberculosis, hepatitis, leprosy, gangrene, viral fever, small pox, measles, mumps, conjuctivitis, etc., the remedies are selected based on their disease symptoms and effect symptoms. The causative phenomena are not considered in these cases. Either the disease symptoms or effect symptoms or both together lead to the simillimum. Hahnemannian totality is derived from the symptoms of all the three spheres (CDE). So, it becomes an arduous and difficult task for beginners to work out a Hahnemannian simillimum. But three-component classification of the totality of symptoms provides a better insight into the Hahnemannian totality. It is observed that even if one or two components of the totality are missing or not pronounced or not perceived, it is possible to reach simillimum by using the third component (either C or D or E) when its essence is available. If more than one component phenomena are available, the case has a strong basis to reach simillimum. If all the three component phenomena are available in a given case, the simillimum is sure to be infallible. But it does not deter us to arrive at a simillimum even if one or two component phenomena are not clearly known, provided the rest of the phenomena have pronounced and characteristic symptoms as essences.

Eventually, the Hahnemannian totality can be viewed to be constituted of a three-component system (e.g. CDE) as follows:

Totality of symptoms ⎡ Causative (C) phenomenon
⎣ Disease (D) phenomenon
⎣ Effect (E) phenomenon

The totality of symptoms can, therefore, be regarded as a system of CDE phenomena. Each phenomenon of the CDE system is strong enough to indicate a simillimum independently provided they are pronounced and characteristic. But each of them may not be pronounced and perceptible in every case of a disease. In some cases, the causative phenomenon may be pronounced, in some other cases the disease phenomenon may be pronounced, while in a few other cases the effect phenomenon may be pronounced. If all the phenomena (i.e. CDE) are pronounced in a case, it is the most ideal situation of finding the simillimum. It is like the worth of gold. But such cases are not frequently observed during clinical practices. However, it can now be stated that the Hahnemannian totality can be classified and systematised into a three-component phenomenon. When symptoms are collected, grouped, analysed and evaluated under these three categories of events, the understanding of a disease and its treatment becomes relatively easy, unambiguous, systematised and well comperhensible.

❖❖❖

CHAPTER-4

Five Outstanding Case Studies

4.1 CHRONIC BODYACHE

A man, Mr. S, aged 28 years, came with a chief complaint of chronic body pain. Sometimes, it is unbearable and makes him restless. He had been suffering from this trouble for last three years. He gets pain in his body here and there. The pain shifts from place to place. He has gastric troubles. He gets acidity, much gas formation and eructation. He has a poor appetite. He prefers sweets and salts. He took a lot of allopathic treatments with analgesics and antacids. He did not get permanent relief. He was on medication for most of the period of his sufferings. During interrogation, he was sobbing intermittently. Tears rolled down his eyes. On being asked why he was sobbing, he opened up his mind. He started expressing his inner feelings. He said that he had been suffering from this ailment (bodyache) for many years now and not getting cured by any treatment. Meanwhile, he got married. Now, he thinks that who will look after his wife if he dies from the disease which remained incurable. Telling this, he started weeping uncontrollably. He has become very much mentally depressed because of long-continued sufferings. He feels that it is better to die than suffering like this. But at the same time he is worried about his wife's future. So, he feels very gloomy and depressed. What I could observe is that his basic complaint was gastric trouble. Much gas formation was the cause of his body pain, here and there. He suffered so much for years together that he developed now a severe mental depression. His constitution was of *Sulphur*. His disease symptoms indicated *Lycopodium*. But he was prescribed two doses of *Aurum mur.* 200C/12 hourly. The remedy was based on his mental symptoms. He recovered very well on *Aurum mur.* He came smilingly after three weeks for a review.

If we analyse this case, we can clearly visualise that his sickness was divisible into three component parts. One can be called the cause of his main disease (i.e. chronic body pain). The cause, here, was the gastric trouble. The second component is the disease itself i.e. his chief complaint (body pain) for which he came for treatment and focused mostly. It was a physical complaint. The third component was the mental effect of the disease and his sufferings. It was a mental depression which I preferred to call an 'effect phenomenon' of the disease. Here, the effect phenomenon was very pronounced and manifested spontaneously to become an essence of the case for remedy selection.

4.2 EPILEPSY

In another case, a young girl, Ms. B aged 19 years, was suffering from epilepsy for two and half years. She used to get convulsion off and on. She was on allopathic medication so far. But the fits returned whenever the medicines were discontinued. During acute attack, she gets unconscious for about half an hour. Frothy saliva comes out from herself mouth during the convulsive attack. She is mentally depressed and introvert and keeps herself aloof from friends. On asking when and how she started getting these fits, her father told that she developed this disorder after sudden death of her mother. She being the youngest of the children was very much attached to her mother. Her disease symptoms indicated *Cicuta virosa*. But she was prescribed two doses of *Ignatia* 200C. This remedy was selected because it was clear that a sudden mental shock due to her mother's death was the cause of the epileptic disorder. This causative medicine did the miracle to cure her complaint. In this case as well, we get three component parts of her sickness. The chief complaint (i.e. disease) is epilepsy, the cause is mother's death and the effect is composed of mental depression, introversion and aloofness. The causative essence, here, led to the simillimum which rescued her from a difficult disease which was taking the toll on her normal life. She was not able to study well, attend college regularly, and socialise with friends. The causative phenomenon was well known here to indicate the simillimum.

4.3 CHRONIC APPENDICITIS

In a third case, a young girl, aged 17 years, came with an acute pain in the appendix region. She suffered occasionally from such pain earlier also. It was a case of chronic appendicitis with an acute flare-up. She was a hot patient. She liked sour, salt and fish. She had much thirst for water. Her stool was constipated. She felt pain on slightest movement and exertion. Her constitutional medicine was *Natrium mur*. But she was given at first *Bryonia* 30C/3 doses/4 hourly and then after a week *Bryonia* 200C/1 dose. She soon recovered from the appendicitis. In this case, her disease symptoms with a peculiar modality led to the simillimum. Of course, *Bryonia* is also complementary to *Natrium mur.*, her constitutional remedy.

4.4 PANIC ATTACK

In a fourth case, a middle aged man, Mr. S, 40 years in age, came with an acute attack of mental tension, anxiety, fear and restlessness. He had a feeling of suffocation in his chest. He felt as if he was going to die. It was a kind of panic attack. On enquiry, it was found that about six months ago one of his friends locked him up in a closed room in a lonely place out of fun. He was sleeping in that room after a lunch. The room had not much ventilation. Even after shouting loudly from inside the room, no body turned up to open the door locked from outside. Neither he could escape on his own as there was not enough big openings in that room in the form of windows or ventilations. In that situation he became very nervous and scared. He felt that he will die of suffocation in the room. His mental shock and fear had been so intense that they have left a deep scar on his mind. Now, whenever he sleeps alone in a room, he suddenly feels that he may die out of suffocation. He wakes up in panic attack. Gradually, he developed a permanent fear and nervousness. Now, off and on, he gets acute attacks of nervousness, fear, anxiety, sweating, restlessness and breathlessness. On analysing the entire situation, it is found that he has developed a permanent fear psychosis which gets accentuated from time to time. It is nothing but a mental effect (i.e. an intense fear of death and anxiety) which was derived as a result of his undergoing a traumatic situation earlier in a locked-up room. So, he was given *Aconite* 200C/1 dose based on the effect symptoms. The remedy cured him permanently. Here, the effect phenomenon was impregnated with the essence of the case.

4.5 SUDDEN FEVER

In a fifth case, I cite here an example of an acute ailment. A small girl child, aged 8 years, came from her school very happily after attending annual sports day. At night around 9 P.M., the child complained of bodyache, lazy feeling, headache, malaise and fever. She demanded medicine from her mother and went into sleep early. On enquiry, it was found that it was a bright sunny day of the summer when she attended the sports activity in the open school ground under the sun for a whole day. Her sudden sicknes was actually due to much exertion in the heat of the sun during sports activity. So, she was given *Gelsemium* 30C/ 3D/4 hourly which was her causative medicine. She recovered very quickly. Here, the causative essence which was very clear guided to the simillimum.

From all the five cases above, it is apparent that all the three categories of events i.e. *causative phenomenon, disease phenomenon* and *effect phenomenon* are equally important in remedy selection. Any one of these phenomena can guide to a simillimum independently and effectively, if the symptoms are pronounced and characteristic in that sphere.

❖❖❖

CHAPTER-5

Causative Phenomenon

5.1 TWO TYPES

For every disease to be initiated there shall be some causative event, agent or phenomenon. It may or may not be apparently recognisable every time and in every case of diseases. But a causative event/agent shall be present behind every sickness, disease or disorder. Broadly, the causative agents/events may be classified into two categories i.e. biological and non-biological. The former includes bacterial, viral, fungal and parasitic agents. The latter includes anything of non-pathogenic causative factors (e.g. physical injury, mental trauma, emotional upset, diet disorder, etc.). If the causative phenomenon is clearly recognisable and correlatable to a disease, the remedy can be selected based on the causative factor. But for each and every conceivable causative phenomenon, the remedies are not yet available in the materia medica. Only those causative remedies which are known in the materia medica are utilised at present. For example, *Arnica* and *Bellis perennis* are well-known causative remedies for effects of injuries, bruises, sprain and blows. I cite here below a few treated case reports.

5.2 CHEEK-BONE TUMOR

Arnica works very well on the soft tissues. *Hypericum* acts well on the nerves tissues. I found *Bellis perennis* to be very effective for both soft and hard (e.g. bony) tissues. I cite here a case study. A middle aged lady, Mrs. K, 35 years in age, had a severe injury of her right cheek bone after hitting the edge of a wooden door in her room. Immediately, she used cold water compresses. Swelling and pain subsided a little. A nearby physician gave her *Arnica* 200C. It gave her futher relief of pain and swelling. After about six months the lady came with a bony tumor on her right cheek. The physician gave her again *Arnica* 1M, then *Arnica* 10M. But the bony growth did not respond expectedly. Then, the patient came for further consultation with me. Since, earlier, *Arnica* high did not work satisfactorily, I gave her *Bellis perennis* 200C/4 D/24 hourly. On a review after one month, it was found that the bony tumor subsided considerably. Then, she was given *Bellis perennis* 1M/3D/24 hourly. After about two months the tumor completely resolved. The causative phenomenon here guided to the simillimum.

5.3 GANGLION

In this case, a high school principal, Mr G, aged 50 years, came with a large-sized ganglion on his left wrist. It was there for about 5-6 years. He was asked how it happened. He remembered that it started to develop after an injury of his left wrist about 6 years ago. The swelling was moderately hard, knotty and moveable. He was given *Arnica* 1M/3D/24 hourly. After three months, he came for a check-up. By that time, the large knotty swelling on the left wrist had completely disappeared.

5.4 SCIATICA

In this case, a lady, Mrs. S, aged 47 years came with an acute pain in her left leg from foot to hip. The pain recurred intermittently for last 10 years. In acute state, she takes allopathic analgesic tablets. On asking about the genesis of her problem, she told that she got this trouble after being deeply injured by an iron nail which punctured the sole of her left foot. So, she was given *Ledum* 200C/3 doses/ 12 hourly. The remedy acted excellently. She was relieved for next three months with least trouble. Then, she was given one dose of *Ledum* 1M. No more acute pain was reported. These are a few examples of causative phenomena utilised for remedy selection. However, these are instances of causative phenomena only at the physical level.

Similarly, there can be causative phenomena at the mental-emotional level. There may be hurt at the emotional level. Then, a sickness may develop at both physical and mental levels. If exact causative factors can be determined in such cases, the simillimum remedies can be worked out. I cite here below a case of causative phenomenon at the mental level.

5.5 MENTAL DEPRESSION

A young girl, Ms. U, aged 19 years, was brought by her mother for consultation. The mother told that for last few months her daughter was having some abnormal behaviours. She did not take food properly. She liked loneliness. She used to weep alone. She did not work properly. She was listless. She was losing interest in her day-to-day activities. On query how it happened, her mother slowly opened up the story behind the scene. The mother told that it started happening after she was deserted by her boy friend with whom she fell in love and whom she wanted to marry. Based on this causative phenomenon, she was given *Ignatia* 200C/3 doses/12 hourly. She recovered completely from this depressive mental state in about one month. In this case, her mental depression was caused by a deep emotional hurt. These are some examples of causative approaches towards homoeopathic therapeutics. In these cases, the causative phenomena could be clearly identified and correlated to the ailments.

5.6 CEREBRAL STROKE

I cite here another interesting case history. A young man, Mr K, aged 35 years, was brought with a complete paralysis of his right side of the body. His right arm, right leg, right face, right half of the tongue were paralysed after a sudden cerebral stroke. He was in semi-conscious state. But he was not able to speak. He had a history of intermittent hypertension. On being asked how it happened, his wife told that he became very angry on some family matters with his cousin and picked up a quarrel. Both quarreled with each other very violently for some time and, then sudenly, he fell down and became almost unconscious. His B.P. was high. The paralytic stroke took place beacuse of an uncontrolled emotional outburst of anger and violence. Based on this causative phenomenon, he was given *Cuprum metallicum* 200C/3D/12 hourly. The remedy brought in a spectacular recovery of his stroke effects. His paralytic condition of right arm, leg, face and tongue started improving significantly from the third day onward. He started walking after ten days and completely recovered in one month.

5.7 COCCYX PAIN

A young girl, Ms. D, aged 16 years, complained of a severe pain in the coccyx. There was no apparent reason for the pain. Her constitution was of *Arsenicum album*. On query, she told that about two months ago she had a fall in the toilet and injured the area of coccyx. Basesd on this causative phenomenon, she was given *Arnica* 1M/1D. She recovered completely and there was no relapse of pain.

5.8 HIGH FEVER

A middle aged Govt. officer, Mr. A, came in one evening with a high fever, bodyache, chilliness, headache and restlessness. He explained that he got this fever after getting wet in the rains during the day time while he was walking on the way to his office. He was given *Dulcamara* 30C/3 doses/4 hourly. The remedy cured him in the night itself. The causative phenomena if clearly recognisable in acute cases can also bring in curative results quickly.

5.9 EXCESSIVE VOMITING

A small child, aged 3 years, was brought by her mother for excessive nausea and vomiting for two days. She was not able to take any food or milk. As soon as she tried to take some food she got vomiting. At other times also, she kept on feeling nauseated. She had no appetite. On query how it all started, her mother could not tell anything significant. But while describing her daughter's sickness she made a pausing remark that the child also vomited a long worm on the first day at noon. Immediately, on this indication, she was given one dose of *Cina* 200C. Within a short time, her nausea and vomiting stopped. From the next day onward, she was quite well with good appetite and health. Here, the intense worm activity was the causative phenomenon behind the child's nausea and vomiting. So, *Cina* did the cure.

5.10 SHOULDER RHEUMATISM

A middle aged man, aged 48 years, came with an acute pain in both shoulder joints. The pain was biting type and made him restless. It was a case of chronic rheumatism for about 5 years. His RA factor was positive. He gets intermittently aggravated pain in shoulder joints and neck. The present acute pain was there for the last 3-4 days. On asking how he got the present pain, he told that this acute pain started when it was raining in the winter night two days ago and the weather became very chilly. The shoulder joints became stiff. He was not able to move his arms due to pain and stiffness. He was given *Rhus tox.* 200C/ 2 doses/12 hourly. The remedy acted very quickly relieveing his acute pain and stiffness. He started improving day by day. The causative phenomenon was the rainy weather which further aggravated the already cold night of the winter to trigger his acute rheumatic pain in the shoulders. *Rhus tox.* was selected only on the causative indication.

5.11 DIARRHEA/DYSENTERY

Recently, after one phase of Polio immunisation programme on 27th January, 2000, many children came with the complaints of diarrhea-dysentry. They had four to five stool a day, changeable in color, greenish or whitish, curd like, sour smelling, also frothy, foamy, gaseous, aggravated towards evening, sometimes leaking without effort. All indicated remedies like *Pulsatilla, Mag. carb., Arsenicum* and *China* failed to relieve them completely. These remedies gave relief only temporarily. But *Thuja* and *Sulphur* when applied on vaccination cause did the complete recoveries of these cases.

5.12 SOME IMPORTANT CAUSATIVE REMEDIES

There are many remedies for non-pathogenic causative spheres. Only some of them are discussed here. For example, injury of nerves may indicate *Hypericum*. The injury of eyes may indicate *Arnica* or *Ruta*. Muscles injury may indicate *Arnica* or *Bellis perennis*. I have observed preventive action of *Arnica* 200C before extraction of tooth. If administered in a few doses, half an hour to one hour before tooth extraction, the medicine prevents incidence of much pain, swelling, bleeding and infection of the gum following the procedure. No antibiotic or hemostatic medicines are needed in such cases. Injury of bones may indicate *Symphytum* and that of head may indicate *Natrium sulph.* or *Acid. sulph.* Punctured wounds may require *Ledum* while lacerated wounds may indicate *Calendula* or *Ledum*. Insects bite may indicate *Apis, Ledum* or *Natrium mur.*

Lodged foreign bodies/splinters/fish bones may require *Silicea, Rhus tox.* or *Laurocearus.* Loss of fluid from the body may indicate *China, Arsenicum, Thuja* or *Natrium mur.* Excessive tea consumption may indicate *Pulsatilla, China* or *Thuja.* Masturbation may indicate *Nux vomica, Bufo, Conium, Natrium mur., Lycopodium* or *Thuja.* Vaccination may indicate *Sulphur, Thuja, Silicea, Kali. mur., Mezerium* or *Malandrinum.* Riding in carriage may indicate *Lycopodium* or *Cocculus indica.* Bad smell may require *Carbo veg.* or *Kreosote.* Drinking beer may indicate *Kali. bichrome.* Milk as causative agent may require *Mag. carb.* or *Natrium phos.* Eating pork may indicate *Pulsatilla, Sepia* or *Natrium mur.* Straining or lifting heavy articles may indicate *Rhus tox., Calcarea carb., Bryonia, Kali. carb.* or *Carbo animalis.* Dentition may require *Chamomilla, Mag. carb., Podophyllum* or *Staphysagria.* Excessive salt eating may indicate *Natrium mur., Carbo veg.* or *Phosphorus.* Eating ices or fruits may require *Arsenicum album* or *Cuprum.* Gas poisoning may require *Carbo veg.*

Alcohols as causative agents may indicate *Opium, Nux vomica, Sulphur* or *Lachesis.* Tobacco habit may require *Argentum nitricum, Tabacum, Arsenicum, Lycopodium, Thuja, Veratrum alb., Staphysagria* or *Acid. sulph.* Radiotherapy may require *Cadmium iod., Radium brom., Okoubaka* or *Phosphorus.* Suppressed menses may require *Pulsatilla, Lycopodium* or *Natrium mur.* Suppressed eruptions may indicate *Sulphur, Apis, Calc. carb., Hepar sulph., Bryonia* or *Causticum*. Poor sleep or night walking may require *Nux vomica, Rhus tox., Sulphur, Kali. carb., Syphilinum* or *Carcinosinum*. A Sun-stroke may require *Natrium carb., Gelsemium* or *Camphora*. An excessive exertion may indicate *Bryonia* or *Rhus tox*. Rain wetting may suggest *Dulcamara, Rhus tox., Arsenicum* or *Malaria officianalis*. Thunderstorms may indicate *Rhododendron, Rhus tox.* or *Syphilinum*. Worm infestation may indicate *Cina, Cicuta virosa, Sulphur* or *Calcarea carb*. New moon and full moon may indicate *Silicea*.

Similarly, there can be causative phenomena at mental-emotional levels. For example, a sudden fear may indicate *Aconite*. A violent outburst of anger may indicate *Cuprum metallicum, Nux vomica* or *Hepar sulph*. A sudden grief may require *Ignatia*. Suppression of emotion may indicate *Staphysagria*. Suppressed anger may suggest *Staphysagria, Natrium mur.* or *Lycopodium*. Apprehension before examination may indicate *Argent. nitricum, Anacardium* or *Lycopodium*. Disappointed love may indicate *Ignatia, Natrium mur., Acid phos., Aurum met., Cactus* or *Veratrum*. Bad news may indicate *Gelsemium, Apis* or *Paeonia*. Fright may suggest *Ignatia, Kali. brom., Lachesis, Aconite, Arsenicum* or *Veratrum*. Anger may indicate *Nux vomica, Lycopodium, Sulphur, Lachesis, Kali. brome* or *Sepia*. Jealousy may require *Apis, Ignatia, Lachesis* or *Natrium mur.*

❖❖❖

CHAPTER-6
Miasm As A Causative Phenomenon

6.1 THE CONCEPT

Miasm is a unique concept provided in homoeopathy by master Hahnemann. In modern terminology, it can be called a genetic predisposition. Practically, it would have been impossible to eradicate many of the chronic diseases without the application of miasmatic (i.e. nosode) remedies, intercurrently. The nosode remedies represent miasmatic susceptibilities of human beings and help to rectify them. Hahnemann recognised three principal miasms i.e. *psora, sycosis* and *syphilis* as fundamental causative factors for chronic diseases. He considered psora to be the oldest and most important of all chronic miasms. It was thought to be associated with all kinds of serious chronic diseases including cancer, diabetes, hypertension, epilepsy, rheumatism and schizophrenia. Bronchial asthma was considered to be due to sycotic miasm. Hahnemann's *pseudo-psoric* miasm was later described as *tubercular* miasm. Koch's infection is considered to be due to tubercular miasm. A chronic ulcer is considered to be due to syphilitic miasm. The chronicity, maintenance and recurrence of chronic diseases are mainly due to two factors:

hereditary susceptibility and environmental influence. The hereditary susceptibility is gene-controlled and transmitted from parents to offsprings. But the environmental influence can be controlled to a large extent by human beings and their activities.

6.2 SIGNIFICANCE

The chronic diseases which are hereditarily controlled pose the greatest challenge to all kinds of therapeutic methodologies. For example, diabetes, primary hypertension, heart diseases or rheumatism are all considered as incurable by the modern system of medicines (i.e. allopathy) because of their genetic control. But in homoeopathy, many of these cases become curable by appropriate long term treatment. The use of nosode remedies intercurrently plays a vital role in curing such chronic diseases. The nosode remedies stop recurrence or frequency of recurrence of a disease, thus cutting short the continuation of the disease and then roll back the disease to eradicate its chronicity. So, we can say that the nosode remedies have capacity to rectify genetic shortcomings and susceptibilities. Hence, the consideration of miasms at some stages of treatment is an essential component of curative therapeutics for chronic diseases. For example, a chronic bronchial asthma cannot be cured without inducting *Tuberculinum*, or *Thuja*, or *Syphilinum* at some stages of its treatment. Similarly, a chronic diabetes cannot be cured without using *Thuja* or *Medorrhinum* at some stages of its treatment. According to master Hahnemann, chronic diseases are never cured on their own. Body's natural defence mechanisms alone cannot cure chronic diseases. If not treated, chronic diseases die only with the death of the subjects affected by them. Therefore, the applications of miasmatic concept and remedies bear a great significance in the whole treatment paradigm of chronic diseases and homoeopathy.

6.3 MIASMATIC SYMPTOMS

Hahnemannian miasms are characterised by some sets of symptoms which clearly differentiate them from one another. Miasmatic symptoms are manifested at all levels of human beings e.g. physical, mental and emotional. They are so characteristic that it is not difficult to recognise them. Fundamental essences of the three main miasmatic groups are as follows:—

(i) Lack of, for psoric miasm

(ii) Excess of, for sycotic miasm

(iii) Deviation of, for syphilitic miasm

For psoric miasm, it may be lack of anything or everything e.g. lack of will power, stamina, initiative, interest, energy, sleep, appetite, heat, fertility, memory, etc. For sycotic miasm, it may be excess of anything or everything e.g. excess of energy, growth, initiative, anger, appetite, sleep, sweat, activity, etc. For syphilitic miasm, it may be deviation, disfigurement, dysfunction, destruction of anything e.g. non-healing ulceration, dystrophy, dysplasia, degeneration of brain cells, deformities of limbs, white discoloration of skin (vitiligo), etc. To further understand the miasmatic symptoms and signals for use in our practice, we can overview the groups of symptoms as given by Dr. P. S. Ortega (1999) in the following table.

	Psoric miasm	Sycotic miasm	Syphilitic miasm
1.	Lack or deficiency	Excess or hyper	Deviation, deformation or destruction
2.	Slow, sluggish (mind, temper, activity)	Quick, rapid, hurried (mind, temper, activity)	Uncontrolled, abnormal (mind, temper, activity)
3.	Atrophy, aplasia	Hypertrophy, Hyperplasia	Dystrophy, Dysplasia
4.	Hypofunction (Physiological)	Hyperfunction (Physiological)	Dysfunction (Physiological)
5.	Irritability (holding back anger)	Irascibility (manifested anger)	Rage (blinding anger)
6.	Weakness of memory	Absent-mindedness	Forgetfulness
7.	Sadness	Grief (expressed sadness)	Prostation of mind
8.	Anxiety (inhibited fear)	Outwardly manifested fear (exaggerated fear)	Anguish (destructive fear)
9.	Inhibition, coldness, feeling of inferiority, lack of fertility, shyness, dryness, impotence, lassitude, weakness of an organ or whole body.	Uninhibited, feeling of superiority, excessively fertile, outspoken, fluency, neoplasm, excessively strong organ or part of the body or whole body.	Indifference, loathing of life, suicidal tendency, abnormal secretion, convulsion, spasm, hemorrhage, putrefaction, destruction of tissues, schizophrenia.
10.	Slow pulse	Rapid pulse	Irregular pulse.
11.	Constipated stool	Loose stool	Irregular stool.
12.	Weakness of extremities	Restlessness of extremities	Ataxia
13.	Inactivity	Hyperactivity	Abnormal activity
14.	Sore, bruised, pressive pain (lack of tone). > from rest.	Stitching, pulsating, wandering pain (instability/hypertone)	Burning, bursting, tearing pain (destructive/disordered pain)
15.	Slow, timid, cold, contemplative, meditative, fastidious, trying to achieve	Impulsive, loud, hyperactive, ambitious.	Revolutionary, anarchist, inciting violence, revenge, hatred, offensive, destructive, absurd, disharmonious.
16.	Dry skin with scales with little or no sweats, unobtainable perfection.	Oily skin with lots of sweating and tendency to form warts.	Skin with ulceration or ulcerative tendency.

According to Banerjee (1996), an anxiety is related to psoric miasm; incoordination (or instability) in behavior/perception and suspiciousness to sycotic miasm; maliciousness, wickedness and destructiveness to syphilitic miasm; discontendedness, displeasure and changeableness to tubercular miasm (pseudo-psoric miasm). Clinically, skin itches are related to psoric miasm; diabetes and hypertension to sycotic miasm; and pleurisy and Koch's infection to tubercular miasm. High susceptibility to catch cold, cough, pneumonia and bronchitis are related to tubercular miasm.

6.4 MIASMATIC APPLICATIONS

Like any other remedies, miasmatic remedies are to be applied on the basis of their characteristic symptoms. The symptoms, signals and indications as shown under para 6.3 provide useful guidelines to the selection of miasmatic remedies. Intercurrent use of miasmatic (nosode) remedies are a must if we are to eradicate chronic diseases. According to Dr. Ortega (1983), when miasmatic symptoms reach surface, their corresponding remedies are to be used. In addition to this, I observed that miasmatic remedies can be used when the principal disease was in dormant state. For example, in case af an allergic asthma, *Tuberculinum* can be used as an intercurrent remedy when asthma is not in active state. Such use of *Tuberculinum* prevents the recurrence or reduces the frequency of recurrence of asthmatic attacks. A chronic disease is continued through its recurrence. When the manifestation of recurrence of a disease is stopped, the disease gets cured. This is the implication of using miasmatic remedies.

I also found *Tuberculinum* to be an effective miasmatic remedy to prevent the recurrence of appendicitis. Similarly, certain other diseases are also cured by miasmatic remedies. For example, I observed in several cases that *Medorrhinum* cured uterine fibroids. *Tuberculinum* cured enlarged, hard, indurated lymph glands of established tubercular origin. So, miasmatic remedies act both as curative and preventive medication. In another case, I observed that *Psorinum* cured bad-smelling, scanty, dark-colored menses in a middle aged woman who had dry, unwashed, shabby-looking skin and hairs and came from a financially poor family background. I also observed that when all indicated basic remedies failed, *Medorrhinum* quickly cured acute attacks of gonorrhoeal infections. Such cases came after the failure of modern penicillin treatments.

6.5 SOME CASE REPORTS

6.5.1 ASTHMATIC BRONCHITIS

A small boy aged 6 years came on 06/03/99 for treatment of his asthmatic bronchitis persistent since childhood. He got frequent cold, cough, sneezing, vomiting, wheezing. He also suffered from constipation and loss of appetite. He was so far under antibiotic treatment from time to time. His coughing and wheezing < at night. He liked sweets, salt, meat. He had a sickly look, bloated abdomen, sallow, pale complexion. His mother told that he was irritable, restless and obstinate type. The basic remedies like *Aconite, Ipecac., Arsenicum, Cina* and *Lachesis* based on disease symptoms falied to cure him permanently. But when his miasmatic medicine which was clearly *Tuberculinum* was administered in 200C potency, the case made a miraculous recovery in a very short time. Here, the miasmatic susceptibility seemed to be the fundamental cause of the disease and responsible for its persistence and chronicity.

6.5.2 LEUCORRHEA

In this case, a young girl aged 20 years came on 12/02/99 for treatment of her chronic leucorrhea. The discharges were thick, white, sticky, VDRL positive. Liked sweets, salts. Stool clear. Menses advanced by 2-3 days and flow normal. Her constitutional remedy was *Calcarea carb*. All indicated remedies like *Pulsatilla, Kali. carb., Sulphur* from time to time could not give her permanent relief. Then, based on a sexual pollution history, the miasmatic susceptibility remedy *Medorrhinum* 200C was administered. The remedy gave her a quick recovery from her white discharges.

6.5.3 CHRONIC SINUSITIS

A young boy aged 15 years came on 30/06/98 for treatment of his sinusitis. He had a thick nasal discharge, nose block, nose pain, headache. He had much thirst, constipated stool. He used to emit a fetid smell from his nose. His constitution was of *Bryonia*. His disease symptomatic medicine was *Kali. Bichrome*. First, *Kali. bichrome* 200C and then *Bryonia* 200C were administered. They gave only temporary relief and could not hold the case for long. But when *Psorinum*, 200C was administered which seems to be his medicine of miasmatic susceptibility, it relieved him permanently. It showed that the miasmatic susceptibility was responsible for chronicity of his sinusitis.

6.5.4 VENEREAL DISEASE

A middle aged man, aged 40 years came on 02/01/98 for treatment of an acute stage of gonorrheal infection. He had a history of pollution of sex 3 years ago and got the venereal infection. His disease symptoms were pain, swelling and burning in the organ and profuse milky white discharge through urethra. He took lots of penicillin treatment, repeated several times during the last three years. They gave him immediate relief but the disease relapsed after some months. He came with an acute pain, burning and thick white discharges which made him very restless, sleepless, anxious and uncomfortable. Based on his miasmatic susceptibility, he was given Medorrhinum 200C. The remedy brought in a miraculous recovery of his condition in a short period.

6.5.6 CHRONIC TONSILLITIS

A young girl, aged 14 years, came on 13/04/99 for treatment of chronic tonsillitis. She had a *Pulsatilla* constitution. She was very mild tempered, preferred sour and salt, had dysmenorrhea. Tonsillitis used to influence on both sides from time to time. It was < during winter season. She had also eyes allergy. Eyes were reddish and used to itch. She was given *Pulsatilla* 200C, then *Lycopodium* 200C and then *Lachesis* 200C over a period of time based on symptoms. But the remedies gave her only temporary relief. Then, on the basis of miasmatic symptoms (e.g. prone to eyes allergy, redness and itching of eyes, dysmenorrhea, aggaravation in cold weather), she was given the miasmatic remedy *Psorinum* 1M. The remedy gave a remarkable relief to her tonsillitis and eyes allergy on a long-term basis. It was apparent from the case that some basic disorder lay at the root of her ailments and it was her miasmatic susceptibility. *Psorinum* 1M when applied removed that susceptibility which was practically the causative factor of her disease.

6.5.7 DOWN'S SYNDROME

A small boy, aged 5 years, was brought for treatment of a serious congenital disorder (down's syndrome) on 12/06/98. He was not able to sit, stand or crawl properly. He was also not able to hold his head steadily. He could not speak clearly. He had excessice salivation. His teeth were badly affected by black caries. He liked much sweets. He was given indicated remedies like *Merc. sol.*, *Cocculus*, *Calcarea carb.* But there was no significant improvement in his condition. Then, based on his excessive anger, profuse salivation at day time, incoordination in the movement of limbs and strong liking for sweets, he was given the miasmatic remedy *Medorrhinum* 1M/3D/6 hourly. In about one and half month, some significant changes were noticed. He could sit properly, crawl properly, but could not yet stand properly. He could hold his head more steadily. It shows that miasmatic remedies possessed potential to improve even some genetic disorders to an appreciable extent.

6.5.8 CATARACT

A lady aged 50 years came on 13/08/98 for treatment of cataract of eyes which was diagnosed by an eye specialist. It was an early stage of cataract formation. She had also eye pain. Her eyesight was weak and vision hazy. Weakness of eyesight used to be < in morning and Sunshine, and > evening and onset of darkness. On these symptoms, she was given the miasmatic remedy *Medorrhinum* 1M. The remedy improved her eyesight considerably over a period of time.

6.6 WHERE TO USE MIASMATIC REMEDIES

Basically, all chronic diseases arise due to constitutional susceptibilities of individuals. For example, a *Sepia* constitution is susceptible to develop cancer of uterine cervix. A *Calcarea carb.* constitution is susceptible to develop gallbladder stone, kidney stone, uterine fibroid, heart disease, uterine cancer, etc. A *Lycopodium* constitution is susceptible to develop hypertension, polycystic kidney, renal calculi. An *Arsenicum* constitution to develop asthma, diabetes mellitus. A *Sulphur* constitution to develop hypertension, allergic rhinitis, anal fissure, skin diseases. A *Phosphorus* constitution to develop tuberculosis, breast cancer. A *Conium* constitution to develop prostate cancer, breast cancer, etc. Similarly, all other constitutional remedies have susceptibilities to initiate some specific chronic diseases. Constitutional remedies are able to recover individuals from many of these diseases in early stage. But miasmatic remedies are needed where the diseases have developed strong chronicity. The miasmatic susceptibilities are responsible for spread, recurrence, persistence and destructive power of chronic diseases. Miasmatic symptoms are manifested for each category of miasmatic remedies. For example, in any fetid discharge, whether from ear, nose, throat, lung, menstrual cycle or leucorrhea, the miasmatic remedy *Psorinum* is indicated. Recurrences and tendencies of most cases of asthmatic bronchitis can be eradicated by the use of miasmatic remedy *Tuberculinum*. A recurrence of bleeding from most cases of uterine fibroids and kidney tumors can be stopped by the greatest sycotic remedy *Thuja occidentalis*. Recurrences of fine, milliary pimples in most teen aged boys and girls can be removed by the miasmatic remedy *Malandrinum*. Similarly, there can be many instances of miasmatic effects on chronic diseases. So, miasmatic susceptibility can be considered as one of the causative factors for initiation, progression, continuation and recurrence of chronic diseases. In many cases, basic remedies work for some time or are not able to cure diseases permanently. Then, miasmatic symptoms can be utilised to use the miasmatic remedy which may be based on the disease miasm or the hereditary background miasm.

6.7 BACKGROUND MIASM AND DISEASE MIASM

In general, every constitution is affected by more than one miasm, active or dormant. But the miasmatic remedies are to be applied based on the active miasm, the dominant miasm or the miasm connected to the principal disease. For example, asthma is basically related to sycotic miasm. But it is possible that in active state of an asthma the miasmatic remedy *Psorinum* may be indicated first. In some later stage, the sycotic remedy *Thuja* can be indicated. Besides this, every individual is under the influence of a dominant miasm in his day-to-day life. It is preferable to call it as background miasm. One's body, mind and emotion are controlled by one's background miasm. This is identified by the general characteristics. For example, psoric miasm is recognised by the characteristics like lack, deficiency or shortage. Sycotic miasm is identified by excess, hyper, over, uncontrol. The syphilitic miasm is known by deviation, destruction, perversion. The tubercular miasm is identified by changeableness, obstinancy, rigidity, cosmopolitanism. Background miasm is inherited. Every individual is born with a background miasm. Other miasms are manifested later as the person grows. For example, after use of multiple sex partners one may develop gonorrhea and the image of *Medorrhinum*, the sycotic miasm. But his background miasm is constant. Temporarily, one can change to another miasmatic influence. But as soon as that influence is over or suspended, the person returns to his background miasm. The background miasm carries his life till death. But in its journey through life, other miasms are superimposed, activated and suspended from time to time. The background miasm shall be either psoric, sycotic, syphilitic, tubercular or cancerous where two, three or four miasms become simultaneously active.

At the present state of our knowledge, it is difficult to further classify the chief background miasms which are hereditarily dominant in individual persons. There will always be an admixture of hereditary miasms in an individual. But we are referring to the dominant miasm of a person in his normal state. Sometimes, it is attempted to refer miasms as *syco-tubercular*, *syco-psoric* or *syco-syphilitic*. This type of classification for mixed miasm may look ambiguous to the beginners. But, here, also the second mentioned miasm is dominant. We have two basic elements in miasmatic analysis. One is the dominant miasm of an individual constitution and the other is miasm(s) of the disease(s) from which the individual suffers. The disease-controlling miasmatic remedies need to be administered at some stage of its treatment to remove the miasmatic influences. At times, it may so happen that the disease miasmatic remedy matches with the background miasmatic remedy. Then, the background miasm remedy is to be applied. Sometimes, the disease miasm symptoms are not clear enough to select a miasmatic remedy. In such situation, the background miasmatic remedy can be administered to remove the constitutional miasmatic influences. Otherwise, the established principle of relationship of diseases and miasms can be applied to select miasmatic remedies. For example, in general, most skin diseases are related to psoric miasm (i.e. *Psorinum*), asthma, diabetes, tumors related to sycotic miasm (e.g. *Thuja, Medorrhinum*), Koch's infection, bronchitis, pneumonia related to tubercular miasm (e.g. *Tuberculinum*), ulcers related to syphilitic miasm (e.g. *Syphilinum*), cancers related to cancerous miasm (e.g. *Carcinosinum*).

To identify a background miasm we have to keep in mind certain symptoms picture which can be more or less representative for a miasmatic constitution. I have observed that the symptoms picture of, or near to *Sulphur* and *Psorinum* can more or less represent a psoric miasmatic constitution. That means that *Psorinum* can be used in such cases as a background miasmatic remedy. Similarly, the symptoms picture of, or near to *Arsenicum album* and *Thuja* can more or less represent the sycotic miasmatic constitution. In such cases, *Thuja* or *Medorrhinum* can be used as background miasmatic remedies. The symptoms picture of, or near to *Cina, Phosphorus* and *Tuberculinum* can represent the tubercular miasmatic background. In such cases, *Tuberculinum* can be used as background miasmatic remedy. On the other hand, the symptoms picture of or near to *Mercurius sol.*, *Aurum metallicum* and *Syphilinum* can be used to detect the background of syphilitic miasm. In such cases, *Syphilinum* can be used as a background miasmatic remedy. For cancerous miasm, the remedy picture of *Carcinosinum* of Dr. D. M. Foubister has enough characteristics to suggest a cancerous miasmatic constitution. So, during the miasmatic evaluation of a subject, it is necessary to evaluate two different fundamental aspects of miasm i.e. (i) background miasm and (ii) disease miasm.

The disease miasm(s) may or may not be a part of the background miasm. Using the background miasmatic remedy, it is possible to moderate some of the angularities, deficiencies or defects in the personality of an individual. It also helps in reducing the disease susceptibilities which are due to the concerned miasm(s). Many a times, we encounter parents asking a physician whether he can do something for their excessively naughty, restless, violent, destructive, disobedient, inattentive, quarrelsome and obstinate children. Homoeopathic answer is a possible 'yes'. Miasmatic remedies in high attenuations do hold some answers to such problems.

❖❖❖

CHAPTER-7

Constitutional Susceptibility As A Causative Phenomenon

7.1 THE CONCEPT

Kent's concept of constitutional remedies is an integral aspect of homoeopathy. Although master Hahnemann talked about physical constitution in his *Organon of medicine*, it was James Tyler Kent who propounded the concept of use of constitution in a major way in homoeopathic remedy evaluation. Permutation and combination of about thirty five thousand genes constitute various human constitutions which are different from one another. Kent's constitution is practically the genetic constitution. Finding similarity of human constitutions to various homoeopathic remedies is an unique approach of treating human diseases. It had been observed by the old masters of homoeopathy that some particular human constitutions were susceptible to some particular types of diseases. For example, *Calcarea carb.*

constitutions are susceptible to become fat, fair, flabby, overweight, develop gallbladder calculi, renal calculi, fibroids, appendicitis, lumbar spondylosis, malignant tumors, hypothyrodism, etc. A *Lycopodium* constitution is susceptible to develop renal calculi, polycystic kidney, hypertension, anal fissure, gout, arthritis, UTI, etc. There can be many such examples. When symptoms of the body, mind and emotion match with those of the remedies, they are found to cure diseases. Broadly, a human constitution is made up of three main elements as follows:—

1. Body (i.e. physical characteristics)
2. Mind (i.e. mental characteristics)
3. Emotion (i.e. emotional characteristics)

When characteristics of these three elements are broadly known in a patient, his constitutional remedy can be selected. But why we approach a remedy from the constitutional angle? It is occasionally observed that a disease does not always manifest its symptoms in prominent and peculiar ways. Neither, the effects of the disease are clearly perceptible or recognisable in some cases. In such situations, the constitutional characteristics of a patient help to determine a susceptible remedy. Through a constitutional remedy, we take a different route to approach simillimum. This remedy works because the constitutional susceptibility probably makes the subject vulnerable to develop that disease. In other words, the constitutional susceptibility is the cause of his disease. So, it can also be called a causative phenomenon for chronic diseases but of different nature.

7.2 FEW CONSTITUTIONAL REMEDIES AND THEIR CHARACTERISTICS

The *Calcarea carb.* type constitution is generally fat, fair, flabby, cold, pale, moist, slow, sluggish, inactive, unsure, polished, delicate, sweaty in palms, waxy in complexion, shy, timid, protective, easily tired, embarrassed, anxiety prone, sympathetic and susceptible to glandular enlargement. The *Nux vomica* type is usually male, intelligent, hyperactive, highly irritable, easily offended, chilly, overworked, mentally strained, highly efficient, working upto late hours of night, demanding high efficiency from others, having some kind of addiction to stimulants e.g. cigarette, alcohol, coffee, rich diet with high-flying life style, suffering from constipation, dyspepsia, headache, piles, prone to short temper, anger and violence.

The *Sulphur* type is stoop-shouldered, quick tempered, selfish, touchy, egoist, proudy, independent, ragged philospher, untidy in habit and appearance, averse to be wasted, having dry and rough skin, sweaty and offensive body smell, redness of all orifices, burning of soles, palms and head, warm bloodedness, liking for sweet and salt, getting easily offended, having tendency to suffer from skin itches and allergies, epigastric discomfort, sleeplessness. The *Arsenicum* type is having thin hands and face, aristocratic look, chilly, restless, very sensitive, neat, tidy, fastidious about dresses and cleanliness, nervous, highly strung, self-centred, perspiring easily and profusely, not-so-ambitious, likes accuracy and details, always feels insecure, great fear of diseases particularly cancer, irritable, artistic in work, always carries a worried espression on the face as if there is a turmoil inside, always having anxiety, takes much care of health, allergic to cold and slight change of temperature, prone to suffer from bronchial diseases, asthma, diabetes, cancer.

The *Pulsatilla* type is usually female, mild, gentle, shy, timid, malleable, romantic, emotional, weeps easily, affectionate, crave sympathy and companions, dependent, bold, gets easily hurt, has varying moods, warm bloodedness, liking for sour, salt and fat, prone to suffer from pre-menstrual tension, dysmenorrhea, hormonal imbalance, breast adenoma, infertility, irregularity in menstrual cycles, cystic ovaries. The *Lycopodium* type is thin, rigid, pale, weak, sickly, sallow, sunken, intelligent, intellectual, looks older than age, having premature lines on face (Nash,1987), head and brain more developed than body, irritable, peevish, cross, ugly, kick and scream when sick, uses wrong words to express and wrong letters to write, weakness of memory, prickly in temperament, miserly, suffers from physical inadequacy, much flatulance, quick satiety, right-sided complaints or right to left complaints, kidney stones, polycystic kidneys, urinary tract infection, right ovarian cyst, bloated abdomen, duodenal ulcer, peptic ulcer, having sour taste, eructation and vomiting, rumbling flatus in abdomen, susceptible to chronic colitis, liver disorder, intestinal disorder, mucus with stool, impotence, prone to shy away from responsibility, has bloated ego (Vithoulkas,1994), cannot tolerate opposition, tendency to dominate over others, bossy temperament.

7.3 REMARKS

Similarly, the characteristic symptoms of all known constitutional remedies are available in various materia medicas. These can be used where constitutional susceptibility is considered to be the causative phenomenon and there is lack of pronounced and peculiar symptoms available in other spheres of sicknesses.

7.4 SOME CASE REPORTS

7.4.1 HYDATID CYST

A small girl child, Ms. S, aged 7 years, was brought on 06/03/99 by her parents for treatment of a large hydatid cyst in the liver. It was diagnosed by ultrasonography on 07/04/98. The size of the cyst was 76x56 mm. The surgeons suggested excision of the cystic growth. The child had poor appetite and a pale whitish complexion. She was lathergic, very fair and little flabby. Her growth was not proper in terms of age. She liked sweets and pork. She was a chilly patient. She was susceptible to cold and upper respiratory tract infection. She had a gland swelling on the right neck. She was slow in studies and sports activity. Her tongue had a triangular red tip. She had history of nose bleeding. No apparent causative factor could be assigned to the disease. It was an internally located disease. No peculiar disease symptoms could be ascertained. Under such circumstances, her constitutional remedy which was *Calcarea carb.* was considered and administered in three doses six hourly. After one month, a repeat sonography was done, which showed reduction in the size of the cyst. The size come down to 49x43 mm on 07/04/99. At every one month interval, USG was repeated to observe the reaction pattern of the medicine. On 19/05/99, the size was 47x38 mm. Again on 31/08/99, it was 37x27 mm. Upto five months the cyst gradually declined in size. After that, there was no more decline in the size of the cyst. There was a halt in the remedial action. Then, *Calcarea carb.* which was her constitutional remedy was again repeated in 200C potency and 2 doses 12 hourly were given. The reduction in size of the cyst again started. It came down to an insignificant size after one and half month. The constitutional remedy here did the miracle. The remedy was considered for the case as there were no other characteristic symptoms to suggest either effect remedy or disease symptoms remedy. Here, the constitutional susceptibility worked as a causative essence of the case. Her constitutional susceptibility was perhaps responsible for the initiation, progression and continuation of the disease. So, the constitutional susceptibility can be called a cause of the disease and so is considered under causative phenomenon.

7.4.2 APPENDICITIS

A young man, aged 27 years, came on 19/06/99 for an acute pain in the right lower abdomen. The Govt. Civil Hospital diagnosed it to be a case of appendicitis. He used to get this pain from time to time over the last few years, and took allopathic analgesic tablets to relieve the pain. There was tenderness over the appendix area. His pain was < from exertion. He also had a chronic headache from which he suffered from time to time. He had much thirst for water, constipated stool and poor appetite. He liked sour, sweet, salt and fish. He was warm blooded. He had mild temperament. No specific external causative factor was found to be related to the disease. Since the disease symptoms were not found enough, he was given his constitutional remedy *Natrium mur.* 200C/2 doses/12 hourly. On a review after three weeks, he showed a complete recovery of the appendicitis. His stool, appetite and health improved much. This is how and where a constitutional remedy was preferred because of the absence of some strong, characteristic symptoms in the disease and effect spheres. It shows that the constitutional susceptibility of *Natrium mur.* subject makes him vulnerable to develop appendicitis. There may also be other constitutionally susceptible remedies for appendicitis. Here, *Bryonia* could also have been considered for the case, which is again complementary to *Natrium mur.*

7.4.3 DIABETES MELLITUS

A bank employee, Mr. S, aged 30 years, came on 31/05/97 for treatment of diabetes. His blood sugar(PP) was 335mg/dl. He was tall, thin, rigid and fair complexioned with sharp nose. Though young, he gradually developed physical weakness. He had frequent thirst for water and frequent and profuse urination. He developed dryness of mouth, nightly urination, 2-3 times. He had clear stool. Appetite was very good. He liked sour, sweet and salt. He was a chilly patient. He was very neat and clean, well-dressed and fastidious. He was a lazy subject. He does not feel much responsibility towards his office work. He likes to do office work only in a routine manner. He had a great fear of disease. He used to feel much anxiety about his sickness. He was a restless subject. He was also self-oriented. The external cause of his disease was not known. The disease symptoms e.g. frequent thirst and profuse urination, nightly urine, dryness of mouth and bodily weakness could not indicate a very specific remedy. These symptoms suggested anything like *Bryonia, Natrium mur., Arsenicum* or *Acid. sulph*. But his constitutional symptoms collectively suggested *Arsenicum album* to be his constitutional remedy. The remedy was given in 200C/3 doses/ 6 hourly. A strict diabetic diet was also advised. His blood sugar became normal in about one month. Then, he was on *Placebo*. After about three months, a mild recurrence of blood sugar was noticed. Then, only one dose of *Arsenicum album* 200C was repeated. It finished the case. Now, it is more than two years. There had been no recurrence of diabetes and no medication, although he had a family history of diabetes mellitus. It shows that the constitutional remedies have the potential to rectify even hereditary disorders on long-term basis. Only a persistent follow-up of the case can reveal whether the disorder (i.e. diabetes)yielded permanently or not. But such cases provide interesting facts about the curative potential of homoeopathic remedies for an incurable and hereditary disease like diabetes mellitus.

7.4.4 EPILEPSY

A young lady, Mrs. A, aged 25 years, mother of one child, came on 08/03/98 for treatment of epilepsy. She started getting this trouble from 11/01/98. She gets the attacks after lying in bed at night before sleep. Seizure persists for 30-40 minutes. She has also a chronic headache (migraine) in the left half of head. She prefers sour, much salt and fish. She has a clean tongue with linear cracks in the middle. She has dark circles around eyes.

Her eyes discharge water from time to time. She is warm blooded. She has less thirst for water and constipated stool. She is prone to quick irritation. No apparent exogenous causative factor could be established. Except the modality, no other prominent disease symptoms could be collected. So, based on constitutional tendencies, she was given *Natrium mur.* 200C/1 dose. Surprisingly, a single dose of *Natrium mur.* cured her case. She was on *Placebo* for six months. There was no recurrence of seizures within this period. It shows that a *Natrium mur.* subject is also susceptible to develop epilepsy. In other words, a *Natrium mur.* constitution indirectly becomes a cause of epilepsy. But it may not be manifested in every case of *Natrium mur.* constitution.

7.4.5 LEUCORRHEA

A middle aged lady, Mrs. S., aged 42 years, came on 25/03/98 for treatment of chronic leucorrhea. The white discharge was profuse and remained same all the time. Her menstrual cycle had stopped for last one year. Earlier, she used to have bad smelling menses. Now, she has headache all the time. She gets sudden flushes of heat, chill and sweating. She complains of burning heat all over the body. Prefers sour, salt and chilies. She has poor thirst, clear stool and intermittent loose stool. She has rumbling sound in the abdomen. Tender in the left lower abdomen. She is warm blooded. She has also occasional burning sensation at the soles of feet. She has a mild temperament. Considering the above-cited symptom picture, her constitutional remedy appeared to be *Pulsatilla*. It was given in 200C/1 dose because there was no apparent causative factor for the chief complaint. The disease symptoms were not enough to suggest simillimum. The remedy gave her a quick relief of the complaint and a scope for further follow-up. The constitutional susceptibility of Pulsatilla was probably the causative phenomenon behind her early menopause, profuse white discharge and hormonal disorder responsible for flushes of heat, chill and sweating. It is also known that *Pulsatilla* is a great remedy to rectify hormonal imbalances, especially in women.

7.4.6 HYPERTENSION

A middle aged lady, Mrs. Z, aged 35 years, came on 29/05/97 to consult for her hypertension. She had also problem of sleeplessness. She had giddiness from time to time. She was prone to mental tension. Her menses was delayed by 7-10 days every month. She had also chronic tonsillitis and difficulty of swallowing food at times. She was warm blooded. She likes sweets and has a history of more salt eating earlier but now has left it due to high blood pressure. Her tongue has a *Rhus tox.* like triangular red tip. She also gets burning of soles from time to time. She is prone to allergic cold, nose block and sneezing. The symptoms suggested her constitution to be *Sulphur*. She was given *Sulphur* 200C/1 dose in early morning, empty stomach. On next visit after one month, her B.P. was found to be 126/88. It is also an example which shows that a constitutional medicine works even in the case of primary hypertension.

7.4.7 PEPTIC ULCER

A middle aged man, Mr. N, aged 45 years, came on 11/07/97 for treatment of his peptic ulcer. It was diagnosed by endoscopic examination. He gets burning and pain in the stomach and chest. Gets < after meal. Sometimes, he gets mucus with stool. He feels very thirsty for water and dryness of mouth. He was a chilly patient. He likes sour/sweet/salt though he does not take sour due to acidity. He is very restless. He has thin hands, long, sharp features and whitish complexion. He was prone to tension and anxiety. He had poor appetite and gas formation. He was very anxious about his disease. He wants to cure it early as he feels that it may lead to some serious disease later on. He was a very fastidious, neat, clean and tidy person. He was well dressed, well spoken, well behaved but a kind of restlessness was visible on his face and in his behavior. He was losing weight. Sometimes, he got sleep disturbance at midnight due to breathing difficulty. He was prone to cold allergy, runny nose, coughing and sneezing. The symptoms picture suggested his constitutional remedy to be *Arsenicum album*. It was given in 200C/ 2 doses/12 hourly. The remedy gave him a quick relief for long time. Though his peptic ulcer developed after a phase of hyperacidity from excessive mental tension and anxiety over his business, his constitutional remedy was able to contain his ulcer and steadily improved his condition from acute sufferings.

7.4.8 UNHEALTHY GROWTH OF HAIR

A young girl, Ms. A, aged 20 years, came on 08/05/99 to consult for her poor growth of hairs. Her hairs were dry, lustreless, split at the tips, short and falling from time to time. She also had dandruff. She had a sickly, lean, thin and dried-up look. She has good appetite but cannot eat full. She has less thirst for water and clear stool. Prefers sour, sweet, oily and spicy food, chilies. She is a chilly patient. She cannot tolerate fan air even in summer. She is prone to cold, cough, sneezing and fever. She is of restless nature. She is even restless while talking, moving, working. She has lack of self confidence and instability of mind. She is indecisive. Even, on the first day of her visit, she only consulted but did not take her medicine. She is suspicious about doctor's abilities whether he or she can cure her. Her menses were late or advanced by a few days. But she has dysmenorrhea on the first day of menses. She has fear of injections, hospitals, operations, medicines. She becomes easily frightened and panicky. She is also impulsive. Her symptoms picture suggeststed *Arsenicum album* to be her constitutional remedy. So, *Arsenicum album* 200C/1 dose/ was given to her to be taken next day morning. On 30/05/99, she came for a review. Substantial changes were visible on her face, skin, hairs and mind. Dryness of hair, color of hair, splitting of hair, fall of hair and dandruff became better. Color, dryness and roughness of face skin improved. Mental restlessness changed partly to a stable state of mind. After one month i.e. 08/06/99, she expressed a little recurrence of complaints. She was given the second dose of *Arsenicum album* 200C. That was the end of all her complaints. After three months, she was a completely different personality. Her hairs have well grown with black, shiny lustre, dandruff gone, cold allergy lessened, hair falling stopped, splitting of hair stopped, health much improved, mind profoundly stablised, self-confidence gained. The whole demeanour changed. Here is seen a miraculous result of constitutional remedy which improved almost all spheres of a human entity where defects and deficiencies were slowly creeping in to create various diseases and an unbalanced personality.

7.5 WHERE TO USE CONSTITUTIONAL REMEDIES

As mentioned earlier, the constitutional susceptibilities, defect, deficiency and disorder are a part of the causative phenomenon of CDE scheme for human sicknesses. These are also a part of the non-pathogenic causative factors. Within the non-pathogenic causes, we can further differentiate causative factors into two groups: *exogenous* and *endogenous*. The exogenous causes are superimposed on the human body from outside. It means that they are environmentally imposed. It may be a physical injury or a life situation or a climatic factor or a diurnal variation or an exposure to an allergic substance. On the other hand, the constitutional remedies are more required for those cases which arise from endogenous causative factors in human bodies. It means the diseases which have genetic control at their roots. Some of the examples are diabetes mellitus, hypertension, vitiligo, spondylitis, heart diseases, asthma, epilepsy, rheumatism, schizophrenia, cancer, Parkinson's, Alzheimer's, polycystic kidneys, multiple sclerosis, etc. These diseases have hereditary factors behind them for their genesis. They cannot be cured without the application of constitutional and miasmatic remedies. Since homoeopathic remedies have not yet been correlated to any specific genes, the constitutional symptoms, whether physical, mental or emotional are fundamental to arrive at a simillimum which matches the constitutional defects, deficiencies and disorders. So, it is essential to look for constitutional symptoms and remedies in these diseases at some stages of treatment even if exogenous causes are known, the disease symptoms are prominent and the effect phenomena are pronounced. That is why the treatment, management and cure of chronic diseases with hereditary control is so complex, difficult, time-consuming and skill-oriented. The treatment needs to be directed towards all three spheres of a sickness (e.g. cause, disease, effect), intercurrently, for permanent recovery, better management or long-term control. I have observed that some cases of primary hypertension cured by constitutional *Lycopodium, Sulphur* and *Natrium mur.* in a single dose of high potency where symptoms matched.

CHAPTER-8

Disease Phenomenon

8.1 THE MEANING

In modern system of medicines (i.e. allopathy), antibiotic drugs are prepared so as to directly encounter the causative bacteria responsible for various types of infectious diseases. On the other hand, homoeopathic medicines have been prepared for use on the basis of manifested symptoms of diseases whether they are caused by bacteria, virus, fungus or parasite. Master Hahnemann (aphorism 6) advised to collect the totality of symptoms from a disease for its remedy selection. His method of totality of symptoms had already been explained in Chapter-2. Dr. Kent suggested to consider generals to particulars for a remedy evaluation. Dr. Boenninghausen's grand symptom (i.e. location, sensation, modality and concomitant) provided another characteristic background for selection of simillimum. Besides these, Dr. George Vithoulkas' essences and Dr. Rajan Sankaran's methods of situational materia medica, central disturbance and delusion help in remedy evaluation and selection.

By a disease phenomenon, I want to mean the sphere of an actual clinical disease and its manifested symptoms although the treatment shall not be based on its clinical diagnosis. For example, a typhoid fever is diagnosed pathologically from a positive widal test. But its manifested symptoms may include: unremittent fever, usually aggravated towards evening, pulse rate disproportionate to body temperature, excessive debility, malaise, loss of appetite, abdominal discomfort, distended abdomen, intestinal tenderness, constipated stool, sometimes nausea or vomiting, thirsty for water or thirstlessness, mild headache, cold feeling in the body, clouded sensorium, etc. There may also be concomitant mental symptoms. The homoeopathic remedy shall be selected based only on the manifested symptoms and not on the causative bacteria responsible for typhoid. If there are characteristic and peculiar symptoms available in the disease sphere, they also lead to simillimum remedy. The disease phenomenon with or without the combination of causative and effect phenomena does have potential to indicate the curative remedy. I cite here a few case examples.

8.2 SOME CASE REPORTS

8.2.1 CHRONIC BACKACHE

Mrs. M.D., aged 40 years, came on 14/07/97 for treatment of a chronic back pain. An X-ray of the lumbar area showed it to be an osteoarthritic spine with chronic disc lesion at L4-L5 level. Back pain was < from any movement. She had also pedal edema. She could not even turn in bed at night because of the back pain. She felt better in rest condition. The pain at times used to spread to her legs. She had constipated stool. Liked sour and salt. H/O Gall bladder calculi cured by homoeopathic medicines. She was given *Bryonia* 200C/3 doses/12 hourly. Gradually, she recovered from the chronic back pain permanently. No further medication was given. The remedy *Bryonia* was indicated by the disease symptoms, particularly its peculiar modality.

8.2.2 LOW BACK PAIN

Mr. S.N.M., aged 38 years, came on 6/7/97 for treatment of low-back pain from which he had been suffering for last 2 years. He had both pain and stiffness in the back. Pain used to be aggravated in the morning after rising from bed on first movement. It was then relieved upto 12 noon. Pain used to be again aggravated in the evening. Pain also moved down the thighs. It was located at L4-L5 level. < cold weather. He liked sweets. He was given *Rhus tox.* 200C/3 doses/24 hourly. The remedy gave him a long-term relief. Here also, the medicine was selected based on the disease symptoms, particularly its modalities.

8.2.3 NOSE BLEEDING

Mr. B.B.P., aged 40 years, came on 17/06/97 for treatment of his intermittent nose bleeding (epistaxis). He had high blood pressure. He also got headache and then nose bleeding. Headache was relieved after nose bleeding. He had right scapular pain. Right nose bled more than the left nose. He liked sour/salt/chilies. He was a hot patient. He was given three doses of *Bryonia*

200C/12 hourly. He was completely relieved of his epistaxis. The medicine was selected based mainly on his peculiar disease symptoms.

8.2.4 RESPIRATORY DIFFICULTY

Mrs. R.D., aged 35 years, came on 30/06/97 for treatment of her respiratory difficulty. She developed this trouble for last three months. She got difficulty in breathing when exposed to dust, smoke, strong smell, cold weather, after little physical exertion, also in sleep, after coughing, after sweating. She liked sour/sweet. She was cold bodily. She felt much weakness after exertion. Her breathing difficulty was relieved by exposure to fan air. She was first given *Arsenicum album* 30C/3 doses/ 4 hourly and then *Arsenicum album* 200C/2 doses/12 hourly. The remedy relieved her quickly. It was selected based on her disease symptoms.

8.2.5 RIGHT-SIDED HERNIA

Mr. H.C.D., aged 30 years, came on 7/7/97 for treatment of a right-sided hernia. He had been suffering from it for the last eight years. He got pain from time to time. Swelling and pain were aggravated when he walked for long, worked hard and did cycling. It was also worse during hot weather. He liked sour/sweet/fish. He was a hot patient. He was given *Bryonia* 200C/3 doses/12 hourly. The remedy slowly improved his hernia on long term. The medicine was indicated by his disease symptoms, mainly modalities.

8.2.6 INTERMITTENT FEVER

Mrs. S.S., aged 21 years, came on 8/6/97 for treatment of a chronic, intermittent fever. She got fever in the evening. Fever < 7 P.M. till she slept. She got burning in the stomach < 3 P.M. Epigastrium and colon tender. Stool constipated. Poor digestion. Gas formation. She was given *Lycopodium* 200C/1 dose. The fever was completely cured over a period of time and there was no more recurrence. The remedy was based on disease symptoms only.

8.2.7 KNEE PAIN

A lady, Mrs. S.D.P., aged 45 years, came with a pain in knees intermittent for one and a half year. Pain < from rest in bed, rising after a long sitting, on squatting position on the ground, cold weather. She preferred sweets. She had mild temperament. She was given *Rhus tox*. 1M/2 doses/12 hourly. She reported after one month a substantial relief of pain. Here also, the disease symptoms (mainly modalities) pointed to the remedy.

8.2.8 HERNIA

Ms. P.K., aged 7 years, came on 21/06/97, with a right-sided hernia. He had constipated stool. Pain and swelling of the hernia < during full moon and new moon. It was also aggravated during cold weather. He was given *Silicea* 200C/2 doses/12 hourly. He was relieved of the complaint over a period of time. The selection of the remedy was based on disease symptoms, mainly peculiar modalities.

8.2.9 COUGHING, FEVER AND HEMOPTYSIS

Mrs. U, aged 30 years, came on 9/7/98 with complaints of coughing for one month and a fever for last 10 days. She had hemoptysis about one month ago. A Govt. Hospital advised her anti-tubercular treatment for 6 months. She had weakness, giddiness, poor appetite. Her blood report showed: WBC =13600, HB = 9.6 gm %, N = 87%, L = 10%, M = 0%, E = 3%, ESR = 129mm. Mantoux test negative. Fever < 7-8 P.M. in the evening. Coughing < 6 P.M. to 10 P.M. till she sleeps. She liked sour/salt. She was thirsty for water. She was given *Lycopodium* 30C/3 doses/4 hourly. She reported back after one week. Fever and coughing subsided. Then, she was given one dose of *Lycopodium* 200C. All complaints were cleared up in about 1 month. Her headache and appetite also improved. The remedy was based on her characteristic disease symptoms.

8.3 REMARKS

In many cases, characteristic symptoms of the disease are pronounced. In such cases, a remedy can be selected based on the characteristic disease symptoms even if the causative phenomenon(C) and the effect phenomenon(E) are not available or clearly identifiable. The modern system of medicines (i.e. allopathy) gives much importance to the disease phenomenon(D). Under this system, the whole treatment is disease-oriented. But since homoeopathy is symptom-oriented, we can use the disease phenomenon only when a disease manifests some pronounced, peculiar and characteristic symptoms indicating an appropriate remedy. Otherwise, the disease symptoms can supplement the pictures of other two phenomena i.e. cause and effect. Master Hahnemann exhorted to collect symptoms from all three spheres of a sickness (i.e. cause, disease, effect) to make his totality of symptoms. But our clinical experiences show that the peculiar and characteristic symptoms from any of the three spheres have potential to indicate simillimum even if such symptoms are not available in all the spheres at a time. In such cases, the symptoms from other spheres can be utilised to supplement, complement, verify or confirm the other poorly manifested sides of a simillimum remedy.

CHAPTER-9

Effect Phenomenon

9.1 THE SYMPTOM EVOLUTION

One physical law of the Nature as enunciated by Sir Issac Newton is that to every action, there is an equal and opposite reaction. Such fundamental law of the Nature is also applicable to a large extent in the case of incidences of human diseases which are dynamic phenomena. Master Hahnemann recognised that a disease was produced as result of interaction between the disease-cause and the vital force of the human body. He identified primary action of a medicine and a secondary action (or reaction) of the vital force of a living organism (aphorism 63). So, the vital force reaction in response to a disease-cause elicits symptoms of a disease at various levels of a human being (e.g. physical, mental, emotional). Thus, the symptoms can be considered as vital force responses at various levels of human body. The vital force is an individualised entity. Its quantitative and qualitative aspects are different for different human beings. Even, it is racially different. For example, the Indians are found to be more susceptible to cardiovascular diseases than the Europeans. The vital force is hereditarily controlled and environmentally influenced. So, its responses to similar causative agents are different in different human beings. That is why, the same virus or bacteria produces different sets of symptoms in different patients. The vital force reactions (i.e. symptoms productions) are also dependent on genetic constitution of a human being. Different genetic types of constitutions react differently to the same stimuli. For example, *Nux vomica* and *Lycopodium* constitutions respond differently to same bacterial infection. Similarly, the vital force reactions shall also be partly controlled by the quantity and quality of the causative agents or stimuli. For example, a mild exposure to an allergic substance may not elicit any prominent vital force reaction (i.e. symptoms). On the other hand, intense and prolonged exposure to the same allergic substance may produce stronger and permanent vital force reaction (i.e. symptoms). The latter shall need medication while the former may not require a medication at all.

9.2 A SUBTLE DIFFERENTIATION

The symptoms are produced by vital force reactions to the disease-causing agents or stimuli. A disease is manifested and recognised by its symptoms developed at physical, mental, emotional and pathological levels. Now, which signs constitute the symptoms of a disease in its true sense and which symptoms are to be considered as the effects of a disease? This differentiation is vital to understand the process of a remedy evaluation and to use various symptoms in their true worth and perspectives for a remedy selection. For example, a fever usually produces symptoms at physical level (e.g. raised body temperature, bodyache, bodily restlessness, poor appetite, costipated stool or diarrhea, thirsty or thirstlessness, poor sleep, vomiting, chill, rigor, burning of body or eyes, coughing, sweating, dryness of mouth and so on). But when a fever produces some prominent mental symptoms (e.g. mental restlessness, anxiety, fear, delirium, delusion etc.), then these may be called the effects of the disease. Similarly, any physical disease can produce effect symptoms at the mental-emotional level. On the other hand, a mental illness can also produce effect symptoms at the physical level. For example, all schizophrenia patients have almost similar mental symptoms but when their physical effects are considered there are variations. The concomitant peculiars at the physical level can also provide clues to the simillimum in such cases. So, the effect symptoms are those which are produced at the levels other than the original level of the disease. The level may be physical, mental, emotional or locational. For example, a mental fear can produce first a mental anxiety, then a mental restlessness, then a sleeplessness, then a hypertension, and so on. So, here, a mental affection (e.g. fear) ultimately produced some physical effects (e.g. sleeplessness and hypertension). In this case, a remedy can be selected either on the causative phenomenon (i.e. fear) or on its physical effects if there are some prominent patterns or peculiarities associated with those physical diseases (e.g. sleeplessness and hypertension). The hypertension may show some kind of rhythmic aggravation or the sleeplessness may show some kind of peculiar time pattern or concomitant symptoms. Sometimes, a physical disease can produce some physical effects at other locations. For example, abdominal gas formation can sometimes cause a chest pain which is often feared as a heart trouble. So, there are different ways as to how a disease phenomenon can be explained, its symptoms analysed, and a remedy evaluated. Mixing up of different symptoms of different levels and genesis together make a remedy picture unwarrantedly complicated and confounded. So, the breaking down of a human sickness into three clear-cut component phenomena and their proper understanding can make homoeopathic therapeutics relatively easily comprehensible, unambiguous and better applicable. Whenever a sickness is encountered by a physician, he can collect and differentiate symptoms into its three main spheres i.e.

(i) CAUSATIVE SPHERE

(ii) DISEASE SPHERE

(iii) EFFECT SPHERE

9.3 DISCUSSION

It seems that the most difficult part of the CDE system is the effect phenomenon of a disease as far as its identification, differentiation, correlation and evaluation are concerned. The effect of a physical disease can be manifested either in the physical or mental sphere or in both the spheres. Similarly, the effect of a mental condition/disorder can be manifested either in the mental or physical sphere or in both the spheres. Thus, it is necessary to differentiate the inherited constitutional symptoms of a patient from the symptoms which have been derived as consequences (effects) of a disease. So, the constitutional symptoms must be differentiated from the effect symptoms. The constitutional symptoms shall lead to a constitutional remedy while the effect symptoms shall lead to an effect remedy. Similarly, the effect symptoms must be clearly separated from the disease symptoms. There is always a scope for a mix-up of the constitution, disease and effect symptoms. But they can be differentiated if closely studied. Then, the remedies can be selected based on the constitutional symptoms, disease symptoms or the effect symptoms. Now, the question arises which sphere of symptoms has to be given more weightage for remedy selection at a particular point of time. This decision depends on various factors discussed later in a separate chapter No. 15.

9.4 SOME CASE REPORTS

9.4.1 TONGUE ULCERATION

A middle aged man, Mr. M, 35 years in age, came on 24/10/9 for treatment of a mild ulceration on the margins of his tongue. He developed it about 1 year ago. He felt some discomfort while eating chilies and spicy foods. More than his physical discomfort, he showed excessive mental anxiety about the disease. He was worried and anxious whether he was developing a cancer. His constitution was of *Merc. sol.* But he was prescribed *Acid. nitricum* 200C/2 doses/12 hourly. It removed his mental anxiety as well as the ulceration over a period of time. The remedy was selected based on the mental effect of his physical disease.

9.4.2 PHARYNGITIS-TONSILLITIS

In this case, Mr. D, aged 46 years, came on with complaints of chronic pharyngitis and tonsillitis. He was suffering from the trouble for last five years. He got intermittent coughing and throat pain. On physical examination, he was found to have granular pharyngitis and enlargement of tonsils with some ulceration spots. Complaints < from any cold exposure, cold water. He was in terrible anxiety. He moved from doctor to doctor for treatment. But getting no permanent relief he came for homoeopathic treatment. He was looking depressed, worried and restless due to an inner anxiety about the disease. He was obsessed with a thought that he was developing a malignancy. His constitution was of *Lycopodium*. But he was given three doses of *Acid. nitricum* 200C/12 hourly. The remedy worked dramatically. He started improving quickly. His mental anxiety had gone. He was a completely different person after a few months. The remedy gave him a long-term recovery. It was selected based on the pronounced mental effect of his physical ailments.

9.4.3 BREAST NODULES

A middle aged lady, Mrs. K, 36 years in age, came with complaints of a few nodules in her breast. One nodule on the left breast was operated by a surgeon. After six months, it started regrowing. Left breast was more affected than the right breast. The nodules were tender to touch, hard, moveable. She showed unusually high mental anxiety about the disease. Sometimes, she rolled down tears from her eyes. She felt that she was developing cancer. She expressed that you must cure her because she had three small children to be reared up. A fear of cancer was deeply rooted in her mind. She had a *Sulphur* constitution. Her disease symptoms suggested *Lachesis*. But she was given three doses of *Acid. nitricum* 200C/12 hourly. The remedy acted miraculously. The nodules started resolving. The mental state of anxiety and worry was much reduced. After one and half month, she was prescribed *Acid. nitricum* 1M/1 dose. No more medication was given. The remedy was based on the effect phenomenon of her physical disease.

9.4.4 CHRONIC GASTRIC TROUBLE

Mr. N.D., aged 48 years, came on 27/7/98 with complaints of chronic gastric trouble. He was intermittently suffering from it for about last 4 years. He was having constipated stool, pain and burning in stomach. Also epigastric tenderness. He liked sweets and salts. He was relieved by drinking cold water. He also later developed prominent heart palpitation, burning of chest and vertigo from time to time. He focussed more on his chest complaints during the interview. His gastric symptoms apparently indicated *Sulphur*. But he was given *Phosphorus* 30C/ 3 doses/ 4 hourly. The remedy acted very well. All his symptoms started lessening. After one week, he was given *Phos.* 200C/1 dose. After one month, majority of her symptoms were gone including the gastric symptoms. The remedy *Phosphorus* was selected based on the effect symptoms of chest which developed following the gastric trouble and he was more focussed on his chest symptoms.

9.4.5 CHRONIC COLITIS

A man, Mr. T, aged 42 years, came on 10/12/99 for treatment of his lower abdomen pain due to chronic colitis which recurred from time to time. On physical examination, the pain was found to be localised in the left colon. He had much gas formation, constipated stool, good appetite but quick satiety. The colon was tender. He liked sweets. He expressed that he felt very weak and tired whenever he was hungry. He cannot tolerate hunger. He had to take food immediately whenever he was hungry otherwise he felt very much exhausted. His disease symptoms indicated *Lycopodium* but he was given *Psorinum* 200C/ 1 dose. The remedy acted well, slowly improving all his symptoms. The medicine was selected based on the peculiar effect symptoms of his body (e.g. a feeling of weakness, tiredness, exhaustion when he was hungry). Thus, the effect phenomenon whether at physical, mental or emotional level can be utilised to indicate a simillimum remedy whenever the symptoms of the effect sphere are pronounced and peculiar.

9.4.6 CHRONIC RENAL FAILURE

Mrs. R.C., aged 33 years, came on 6/8/98 with a diagnosed CRF. An USG on 27/7/98 showed bilateral renal parenchymal lesions. Both kidneys have become smaller in size. Right kidney = 75 mm x 33 mm and left kidney = 76 mm x 37 mm. Urine albumin ++. Pallor +++. B.P. 160/110. Hb = 7.5 mg %. Blood urea = 59 mg/dl. Creatinine = 1.8 mg/dl. Urine output reduced but frequency was more. Edema of feet. Face swelling < morning. She had poor appetite, constipated stool, much thirst for water, headache, tasteless tongue. Got very exhausted on little walking. Bodily hot. Felt very weak physically. The disease (renal) symptoms were not peculiar and pronounced enough in the case. On the other hand, the renal disease had pronounced effect on the alimentary tract, blood pressure (e.g. hypertension), physical strength (e.g. excessive debility) and fluid distribution (e.g. edema,) etc. All the effect symptoms when put together indicated *Acid. mur.* (combining Acidum and Muriaticum). So, the remedy *Acid. mur.* 200C/3 doses/12 hourly was given. The remedy worked very well to relieve the patient for a long time.

9.4.7 HYPERTENSION

A lady, Mrs. M.S., aged 42 years, came for treatment of her hypertension. She was on allopathic medication for three years. She now got trembling of her whole body at times. Left side of her head felt much heavyness. Her left eye discharged water. Her left abdomen had rumbling sound from time to time. Her left colon was tender. She often lost control of her temper. She felt weakness in her left chest. She liked sweets. Her B.P. got aggravated whenever she worried about her family matters. Her disease (e.g. high blood pressure) symptoms were not peculiar in the case. But the effect symptoms when combined indicated *Lachesis* which was given in 200C/2 doses/12 hourly. It brought down the hypertension to normal level over a period of about one month. There were also fat and salt restrictions in her diet. In general, we consider the above symptoms as concomitants, but in differential sense these symptoms constitute an effect phenomenon.

9.4.8 PANCREATIC CANCER

A middle aged man, Mr. K.L., aged 42 years, came on 17/5/97 with an advanced malignancy. Primary tumor was in the pancreas. There were also multiple secondary tumors in the liver. It was diagnosed as poorly differentiated carcinoma. He came after 5 doses of chemotherapy at Guwahati. No radiotherapy was given. He had poor appetite, poor digestion, constipated stool, yellow urine, obstructive jaundice, extreme tenderness of liver, epigastricum and colon, very clean and shiny tongue, pain in the right scapula. Pain < 4 AM to 10 AM. He was given on the first day *Chelidonium* 30C/3 doses/ 4 hourly. After two weeks he reported to be quite relieved of many of his discomforting symptoms. He was then given *Chelidonium* 200C/1 dose. The remedy maintained him well for several weeks although the case was in the terminal stage. The remedy was selected not on the basis of his chief disease (i.e. malignant tumor) or constitution or miasm but on the effect symptoms of the body, which were pronounced and characteristic.

9.4.9 DIABETES MELLITUS

A lady, Mrs. S, aged 45 years, came on 30/12/99 for treatment of diabetes from which she had been suffering for the last 2 years. She was on allopathic Daonil tablets. Her blood sugar (PP) was 400 mg/dl and urine sugar +++. Her constitution was of *Calcarea carb*. She had frequent urine, not much thirst, good appetite, bodily weakness. Most prominent symptoms were excessive leg pain and back pain. She could not sleep at night due to leg pain and a feeling of restlessness in the leg. She was focussing more on these symptoms during interview. She was given *Rhus tox.* 200C/3 doses/12 hourly. After 15 days, the blood sugar (PP) came down to 237 mg/dl. Then, she was on *Placebo.* After one month, BS (PP) was 190 mg/dl. Here, also, the remedy was selected based on the effect symptoms of body, which were very pronounced. The physical disease produced here a pronounced effect at the physical level.

9.4.10 FISH BONE INJURY

An old lady, Mrs. R, aged 58 years, came on 20/01/2000 with a complaint of throat pain. She told that she had a fish bone stuck up in the throat about one and a half month back. She took lots of medicine including homoeopathic medicines (e.g. Ledum, Silicea). But her pain sensation did not subside totally. No fish bone was seen in the throat on physical examination. But, now, she had developed an intense fear about the throat pain which she could feel during empty swallowing. She expressed an underlying fear of cancer. She wanted to know whether she was developing a cancer. She was prescribed *Acid. nitricum* 200C/2 doses/12 hourly. After 15 days, she came smilingly and reported that her throat complaint had completely gone. The remedy was purely based on the mental effect of the physical disease. The effect phenomenon at the mental level was very pronounced. She was almost obsessed with thought of fear, anxiety and worry about the throat pain which she felt might turn into a cancer. Here, the disease symptoms had no peculiarity. The causative medicines (e.g. *Ledum, Silicea*) also did not work. But the effect symptoms of mind did the result. Some may say it is a concomitant mental symptom. It is true. But, in true sense, it was the mental effect of her physical disease.

9.5 REMARKS

From the study of case reports as discussed in various Chapters i.e. 5, 6, 7, 8 and 9, it is now clear that the cause, disease and effect phenomena of a sickness are fundamental to a remedy evaluation. The characteristic symptoms may or may not be manifested in all the three spheres of a sickness at the same time. But a simillimum can be found based on the phenomenon where lie the pronounced and peculiar symptoms. I cite here three short case reports to further exemplify this fact. A lady, Mrs. J, aged 40 years, came on 05/09/99 for treatment of diabetes with blood sugar (PP) = 357 mg/dl. Her urine, appetite and thirst for water were not much significant. But she told that she was having a severe constipation, much irritability, cold feeling and poor sleep at night. She did not pass stool for last 5 (five) days. Based on these symptoms she was given *Nux vomica* 200C/3 doses/12 hourly. After two weeks, her blood sugar (PP) came down to 212 mg/dl. Here, the medicine was selected based on the effect symptoms of body and not on her disease (diabetes) symptoms. In a second case, a lady came on 03/01/2000 with eczema in her legs and hands. She was suffering from the disease for about three years. It was a dry-type eczema with itching and scaling from time to time. But in summer, it used to form pustules and little discharges. She took lots of allopathic medication and used many ointments. On query that in which location she first had this disease, she remembered that she first got it in her legs and then after some months it spread to her hands. Based on this peculiar movement (upward) characteristic of the disease, she was given *Ledum* 200C/2 doses/12 hourly. The remedy worked for months together slowly improving and clearing her eczematous patches. Here, the remedy was selected based on a peculiar disease symptom.

In a third case, a lady, Mrs. S, aged 47 years came with a pain in the left side of her body from foot to hip. On query that how she got it, she said that she started to get this pain after an injury by a nail at the sole of her left foot about 10 years ago. Based on this causative phenomenon, she was given three doses of *Ledum* 200C/12 hourly. In one month, she had substantial relief of her pain and discomfort. Then, after three months one dose of *Ledum* 1M was given. These cases only demonstrate that each and every case of sickness can be analysed perspectively from the point of view of *cause, disease and effect phenomena*. These phenomena can be clearly differentiated in each case and the simillimum remedy can be selected based on the observations from the three spheres. Here, we are only identifying and correlating the facts of the manifested symptoms. There are no extrapolation, imagination, interpretation or ambiguities. We are using only the facts as told by a patient and his companion and observed by the physician as they are. So, these are true representations of three main component parts of a sickness. The numbers of symptoms observed in each sphere are insignificant. The importance lies in the true representation of each phenomenon (i.e. cause, disease and effect) for every case.

From these observations, it can emerge that, basically,

homoeopathy is not an art. It can be an art of healing. There is no art in the remedy selection. It is made out to be so by some. It is only the hard facts which decide a remedy selection. If we want to consider the remedy selection as an art, we shall introduce many elements of ambiguity, uncertainty and interpretation into that process because the art has an unlimited scope of imaginations. In every disease which is a natural phenomenon there are clear-cut symptoms which are to be identified, differentiated and systematised into three components (i.e. cause, disease and effect) for their proper evaluation. The value or worth of each phenomenon are to be decided based on the clarity of symptoms, prominence of symptoms, quality of symptoms, peculiarity of symptoms and patient's focus of symptoms. Then, either an individual phenomenon or a combination of two or three phenomena can be utilised to select the simillimum. The remedy selection, thus, becomes a fact-based, systematic, characterised and unambiguous procedure of working out similarity of a medicine with a disease/disorder.

✤✤✤

CHAPTER-10

Genes And Miasms

10.1 HEREDITY AND DNA

The process of transmission of biological characters from one generation to another is known as heredity or inheritance. And the study of understanding of biological properties which are transmitted from parents to offsprings is called genetics. G.J. Mendel (1865) was first to present to the world the laws of inheritance. Every generation of every species resemble its ancestors. The process of heredity plays an important role in the formation of a new generation. The fundamental hereditary biological units which are a part of this process and transmitted from parents to offsprings are known as genes. A gene can be called a large chemical radical of elements like carbon(C), oxygen(O), hydrogen(H), phosphorus(P) and nitrogen(N) attached to undifferentiated proteins-cum-thread called chromosome. The chemical molecular entity of a gene is called DNA (deoxyriboneuclic acid) which has a double helical structure. The double helical structure of a DNA molecule is composed of nitrogenous bases joined by deoxyribose pentose sugar which is again linked to phosphate compound (i.e. phosphoric acid). The nitrogenous bases are joined through hydrogen (H) bonds.

10.2 GENES AND ENVIRONMENT

The genetic constitution of an organism is known as genotype whereas the expression of observable structures and functional traits is called phenotype. The phenotype expression includes body, form, color, sex and behavior produced due to interaction of the genes and the environment. Homoeopathic constitutional remedies of Dr. Kent practically include both the genotype and phenotype characteristics. Some molecules like vitamins, hormones, metal ions, chemicals and pathogens can induce or repress genes. These are how environment can affect gene expressions and cause diseases in human beings. It was Charles Darwin(1859) who was first to propose the theory of natural adaptation. According to him, the natural environment acts upon the hereditary variability of a species to preserve only those individuals which are better adapted to it. A disease can be taken as a failure of adaptation to the environment. So, it is both nature and nurture which affect the growth, development and differentiation of an organism. In terms of genetics, mutations are the sources of all kinds of variations in human beings. The mutation is a sudden, stable, discontinuous, inheritable variation which appears in an organism due to a permanent change caused in its genotype. When a gene mutation involves deletion, insertion or substitution of a single base pair, it is called point mutation. When a mutation involves more than one base pair or entire gene, it is called gross mutation.

10.3 HUMAN VARIATIONS AND MUTATIONS

Mutations are responsible for developing new traits in a human race. In some genes, the rate of mutation is very low while in some other genes it is very high. Also some genes mutate more frequently than other genes. Various permutation and combination of characters of genes produce varieties of human constitutions. That is probably the reason we find a large number of different homoeopathic constitutional remedies in the materia medica. But the sum total characters in a population remains same. That is why, in materia medica, it appears that as if all the remedies have almost similar symptoms and many of the symptoms are common among the remedies. Since there are a large number of genes (i.e. about thirty five thousand) in human beings, it is obvious that there shall be a large number of human constitutions because of a large variety of mutational variations. That may be the reason why we do not find 100% match of total symptoms in the known remedies of materia medica.

10.4 MIASMATIC DOCTRINE OF HAHNEMANN

It was the astounding genius of master Hahnemann (1812) who introduced the miasmatic concept in homoeopathy about half-a-century before Darwin (1859) and Mendel (1865) pronounced their theories of natural selection and heredity respectively, finally leading to the evolution of modern molecular biology and genetics. Hahnemann (1812) in his *Organon of Medicine* clearly mentioned about heredity and environmental influence on human health. His miasmatic doctrine developed after practical observations that many of the human diseases kept on recurring in spite of adequate conventional treatments. Two principal reasons were thought for this kind of phenomenon. First requirement was heredity and the second requirement was the effect of environmental factors. According to Hahnemann, the second element included incorrect suppression of acute diseases. When initial manifestation of a disease was not correctly or completely cured, the disease became more deep-seated and persistent giving rise to its chronic nature. For example, most skin diseases when suppressed through external application of ointments, they disappear temporarily only to return after some weeks, months or years. Similarly, when chancre diseases are initially suppressed by the application of modern medicines, they become more deep-seated and chronic. So, for a disease to become recurrent and chronic, Hahnemann visualised three fundamental predisposing factors which he termed as chronic miasms. He described them as psoric, sycotic and syphilitic miasms. So, the miasms are practically the genetic susceptibilities which the modern molecular biologists describe to explain the evolution of serious chronic diseases. For example, the gene P 53 is found to be responsible for majority of cancers, CDK4 for melanoma skin cancer, BRCA1 and BRCA2 for breast cancers, B27 for spondylitis, DR2 for tuberculosis, etc.

10.5 MIASMATIC SUSCEPTIBILITIES

It is now clear that Hahnemannian miasms are related to the modern concept of genetic susceptibilities. In the present day when technological advancements are of very high order, the geneticists are able to identify a number of specific genes which are responsible for some specific diseases. But in those days of almost non-existent technological support, Hahnemann could conceive not only the basic susceptibilities of human beings to diseases but also their true nature. The introduction of the concept of miasm was no less an extraordinary feat than the discovery of homoeopathy itself. The basic susceptibilities which developed due to association or suppression of skin diseases (i.e. itch) were called psoric miasm. The susceptibilities which were acquired due to association or suppression of gonorrhoeal diseases were called sycotic miasm. The susceptibilities which developed because of association or suppression of chancre diseases (syphilis) were called syphilitic miasm. Therefore, the basic idea that the disease susceptibilities developed in human beings because of an interaction between the hereditary and environmental factors was described by master Hahnemann as long as more than 50 years before the advent of genetic concept of Mandel(1865). The same phenomenon of interaction is strongly valued by the present day geneticists for the causation of diseases. Hahnemann grouped the entire range of diseases under those three categories of miasmatic susceptibilities, the symptoms and signals of which have already been described in chapter 6. Though it was a broad classification of diseases and their genesis, it was highly technical because of its derivation from the years of practical experiences and support by a large number of manifesting symptoms at all the levels of a human being (e.g. physical, mental, emotional). The manifesting symptoms indicate the basic susceptibilities. Hahnemann also suggested medicines for those miasmatic susceptibilities. For example, *Psorinum* and *Sulphur* for psoric diseases, *Thuja* or *Medorrhinum* for sycotic diseases, and *Syphilinum* for syphilitic diseases. During the treatment of chronic diseases, the application of these nosode remedies became almost essential.

10.6 INDUCED MUTATION: AN EXAMPLE OF ENVIRONMENTAL INTERACTION

The spontaneous mutation rates of genes are very low in all locations of human body. But there are physical and chemical agents which can induce much higher rates of mutation and stable changes in the genes (i.e. DNA molecules) causing various diseases. Such agents are called mutagens which disturb the replication, transcription and translation mechanism of DNA. For example, X-rays or gamma-rays produce ionizing effects on the DNA molecules. They distort or break DNA duplex structures, disturb replication mechanisms and alter gene activities which control normal growth and development of human cells. Almost every chromosome bears oncogenes (i.e. cancer-causing genes) but they remain repressed and carry on normal activities when they are called proto-oncogenes. But when they loose their cell control mechanism, they stimulate excessive and uncontrolled cell divisions. Such cells lack normal properties of cell surface and continue to divide to give rise to the masses of tissues called malignant tumors. The mutagens which cause cancers are known as carcinogens. Some examples are: tobacco products, cigarette smoke, products of hydrocarbons (e.g. petroleum, coal), some metals (e.g. aluminium, nickel, cobalt, arsenic), nuclear radiations, etc. Some viruses (e.g. human papilloma virus) are also found to cause cancer especially in the female uterine cervix. These are only some of the examples of interactions between the human cells and environmental agents to cause human diseases.

Cancer, in terms of molecular biology, is an excessive and uncontrolled growth of malignant cells. In parallelism, in homoeopathy, an excessive growth symptoms or hyperactivity are included under the category of sycotic miasm. So, a cancer is initiated, promoted and progressed under the influence of sycotic miasm. In modern genetics, cancers are initiated, promoted and progressed by cancer-susceptible genes e.g. P53, BRCA 1, BRCA 2, CDK 4, etc. So, in molecular biology, it is the susceptibility gene while, in homoeopathy, it is the susceptibility miasm which are responsible for the cause of a chronic disease. The sycotic miasm has even a larger connotation because it includes all the diseases which show the symptoms of excessive activity manifestations in addition to those of cancer. For example, clinical diseases like diabetes, hypertension (high blood pressure), asthma, etc., are all examples of sycotic diseases although the causative genes responsible for all of them are different. So, an individual Hahnemannian miasm (e.g. psoric, sycotic or syphilitic) shall include a large number of causative genes which are responsible for clinical diseases having affinity to 'lack', or 'excess', or 'deviation/destruction' characteristics. For example, an advanced or terminal stage cancer destroys the tissues and organs of human bodies. So, such a destructive stage where genes have gone completely haywire is known to be under the influence of syphilitic miasm. At present, there is only palliative therapies available for such destructive stages of gene or miasmatic activity.

10.7 INHERITED MIASMS AND ACQUIRED MIASMS

The inherited miasms are susceptibilities provided by the genes and chromosomes which have been transmitted from parents to offsprings. On the other hand, the acquired miasms are susceptibilities which have developed due to changes in the heredity genes (i.e. DNA molecules) by interaction with the environmental factors e.g. certain chemicals, hormones, radiations, pathogens, etc. These acquired changes in the gene structures are again transmitted to the next generation of an organism. This is in some way comparable to the *'roots of diseases'* of Dr. Rajan Sankaran(1997). The susceptibility which is transmitted through gene transfer from parents to offsprings can be called hereditary miasm. On the other hand, the miasm which is acquired as a result of interaction between the genes and the environment can be called acquired miasm. Formation of a malignant disease can exemplify this phenomenon. For example, we know that almost every chromosome bears cancer-causing genes known as oncogenes. In general, such genes remain in repressed (i.e. inhibited) state as far as the initiation of cancer is concerned. At that stage, these are known as proto-oncogenes. A constant physical irritation of tissues of lungs by excessive smoking can induce such proto-oncogenes to loose their normal function and stimulate uncontrolled mitotic divisions to form malignant tumors. Once the malignancy has formed, it becomes an acquired miasm. So, here, the miasmatic susceptibility of cancer has developed for the next generation of organism. For the present generation, it is an acquired miasm while for the next generation down the line it becomes an inherited miasm.

10.8 GENE EXPRESSIONS AND HOMOEOPATHIC CONSTITUTIONS

There are about 35000 genes in human organism. But all the genes on chromosomes are not expressed simultaneously. The cell permits expression of only some of the genes at a time while keeping other genes repressed or inhibited. The repressed genes can be activated either by some metabolic requirements or by some external agents which can interact and alter gene activity. There are a large number of human constitutions in terms of genotype and phenotype characteristics. Such large variations are due to the presence of a large number of human genes, their regulations, expressions, mutations, environmental interactions, apart from chromosomal characteristics and their mutations. So, it is a complex phenomenon which is responsible for such a large variability in the characters of human population. Compared to this large variation, our homoeopathic constitutional remedies in the materia medica are limited in numbers. At the same time, the known constitutional remedies also do not match 100% of the symptoms and characteristics of an individual human. In reality, a 100% matching of similarity is not possible because the genotype and phenotype characters of a person have been so much differentiated by his hereditary and environmental factors from generation to generation. The controlling factors and their influences are so diversified that we can never achieve a 100% similarity of a remedy in a human constitution which is Nature's creation. Because of this fallacy, we observe manifested symptoms at different levels, of different qualities, and in different quantities. Consequently, no two humans are found to be exactly similar in their entities.

The greatest implication of the presence of a large variation of biological characters of human population and a lack of 100% match of similarity between the remedies and the human constitutions is that man is mortal and destined to die. And therapeutically, the implication is that a large number of remedies shall be required to treat human constitutions and diseases.

10.9 GENOTYPE/PHENOTYPE AND THEIR IMPLICATIONS IN REMEDY SELECTION

It is known that gene is a hereditary factor which determines the biological characters of organism. It is inherited and remains unchanged unless severely affected by an environment. The phenotype is the expression of observable structural and functional characters produced due to interaction of the genes and the environment. The different phenotype usually have different genotypes. For example, *Calcarea carb.* and *Arsenicum album* have both different phenotype and genotype characteristics. *Calcarea carb.* phenotype shall usually have fat, fair, flabby, overweight, physical build-up. *Arsenicum album* phenotype shall usually have thin hands, face and eye lashes with aristocratic look. The *Calcarea carb.* genotype is normally slow, sluggish, mild, soft, shy, timid, compassionate, lacking self-confidence, lacks decision-making abilities, has fear of diseases particularly of heart diseases and cancer. The *Arsenicum album* genotype is usually quick, restless, anxious, irritable, fastidious, self-oriented, always feels insecured, lacking ambition, shies away from responsibility, fear of infections and diseases particularly of cancer. Kent's first grade generals usually belong to the genotype characteristics while the second and third grade generals including the particulars usually belong to phenotype characters. The genotype, phenotype and some peculiar concomitant symptoms generally constitute Hahnemannian totality. On the other hand, the genotype and phenotype characters together suggest Kent's constitutional remedies. Since genetic (i.e. gene) constitutions remain unchanged, the genotype characteristics shall be of highest values in homoeopathic remedy selection. The phenotype characters which may change under the effects of environment are next in importance in any remedy evaluation. Apparently similar-looking phenotypes may have different genotypes. That is why, all fat-fair-flabby looking constitutions are not *Calcarea carb.* in genotype. So, it is necessary to probe into the genotype characters of human constitutions for selection of simillimum remedies.

10.10 DOMINANT AND RECESSIVE CHARACTERS OF GENES AND THEIR IMPLICATIONS IN HOMOEOPATHY

According to Mendel, the dominant characters of genes will be inherited by 75% of the offsprings. In other 25%, these characters will recede into the background and other traits will reappear. The dominant and recessive forms are present in the ratio of 3 : 1. That is why we possibly observe polarities in homoeopathic remedies. For example, in majority of the genotypes of a remedy (e.g. *Nux vomica*), we observe dominant characters of that remedy (e.g. irritable, hardworking, efficient, addicted). At the same time, we also observe in a few cases apparently contradictory characters of *Nux vomica* (e.g. mild, lazy, underactive type). This is due to recessive form of dominant characters of genes in a minority population of *Nux vomica*. Practical observations have been made in the past on the existence of polarities of homoeopathic remedies by various learned physicians (e.g. *George Vithoulkas*). But, now, we can find an explanation of such homoeopathic phenomena in terms of molecular biology and genetics. The polarities of remedies are genetically controlled. In clinical practice, the difficulties are faced when we encounter the recessive form of a remedy. In such cases, finding out of Hahnemannian totality can be most appropriate way to reach simillimum because it embodies all the characters (i.e. symptoms), genotype, phenotype, strange, uncommon and peculiar, in a subject.

10.11 REMARKS

It is ironical that often one physician becomes highly critical of another for his suggested methodology of remedy selection. It becomes almost meaningless when we look critically at the complex inner variabilities of the Nature's creation of human beings. Every individual presents us a large number of characteristics in a large number of ways, both quality- and quantity-wise. It is upto a physician what characters and expressions he collects and how he considers, analyses, evaluates and synthesises into a remedy picture of a subject. If it is logical and finds successful and universal application in the treatment of human diseases, it is to be considered. What we do or achieve is only an approximation to the totality of characters (or symptoms) of an individual patient. A homoeopathic simillimum can be considered as a best-fit approximate remedy. Some may arrive at the next similar remedy. Some others may arrive at a near-similar remedy. All can relieve a disease but in different frameworks of time. The remedies other than the best-fit remedy (i.e. simillimum) may take a little longer time and a little longer route which may require a number of successive remedies in the process of a cure. As such also, a long standing chronic disease cannot be cured by a single remedy in most cases.

※ ※ ※

CHAPTER-11

Speed Of Symptom Evolution And Its Implications

11.1 SOME TENETS OF LAW

The principle of similia similibus curentur is the foundation of homoeopathic treatment. It is clearly enunciated in aphorism 27 that the curative power of a medicine depends on how much similarity of symptoms it possesses to that of the disease (Hahnemann, 1994). Although it is broadly known that acute diseases develop fast and chronic diseases slowly, it is not specifically known at what pace the symptoms evolve during the course of a disease. George Vithoulkas states that in acute diseases we may even require a large number of remedies one after another if indicated. Similarly for cure of chronic diseases, Master Hahnemann says, a number of remedies may be required if symptoms change successively for various remedies one following another. A systematic treatment follows in ladder-like steps with the change of symptoms (Burnett, 1989). All these statements of great masters of homoeopathy do have profound implications on the homoeopathic treatment procedures. This is exemplified here below by a short case report of a duodenal ulcer which I had an opportunity to treat.

11.2 THE CASE REPORT

A middle aged person, Mr. D, aged 42 years was presented with an acutely exacerbated state of duodenal ulcer on 6th November, 1996. The ulcer was diagnosed by an allopathic physician from Ba-meal X-ray. He was having a violent stomach pain and vomiting for the last two days and was under allopathic medication. But since the treatment could not stop his recurrence of pain and vomiting completely, he was brought for homoeopathic treatment. On presentation, he had an agonising stomach pain and severe vomiting. Since he came after a just-concluded allopathic treatment, he was given one dose of *Nux Vomica* 6C. On waiting for about five minutes, his symptoms completely changed. He became extremely restless from pain and was rolling from side to side in the bed, asking for drinking water at short intervals and vomiting watery fluids. Based on these symptoms, he was immediately given one dose of *Arsenicum album* 30C. Within minutes, his condition started improving. His pain considerably subsided, vomiting stopped and he became quiet. But, surprisingly, after another fifteen minutes, his symptoms further changed. He suddenly got up from the bed, sat on his legs with knee-chest position, and was pressing hard his abdomen with the hands and folded legs. When asked about why he was sitting like this, he told that he got relief of his pain on sitting at this posture. Based on this peculiar symptom he was immediately given one dose of *Colocynth* 200C. The remedy remarkably relieved his condition. After waiting for about half an hour, he went home walking on his own without any support from others. No more medicines were given except *Placebo*. There were no report of recurrence of symptoms.

11.3 ANALYSIS OF THE CASE

This case is an amazing example of how symptoms and remedies can change so speedily in acute diseases. In such case of a disease which is fast evolving, the change of a remedy is essential whenever evolving symptoms demand it to match the disease course. This way ensures a faster recovery. The case also corroborates the applicability of Dr. J. C. Burnett's third principle of trinity that is every remedy has its own *'range of action'*. *Nux vomica* though was empirically applied, it opened up the case to give rise to *Arsenicum*. The *Arsenicum* when employed acted well but it had a short range of action and gave rise to the state of *Colocynth* which finished up the case. Progressive action of a series of three remedies quickly resolved the case. One may ask if *Colocynth* could have been given at the first instance, or could one remedy have cured the case ? But there were no characteristic symptoms similarity for *Colocynth* to be given in the beginning. The *Colocynth* symptoms developed only after *Arsenicum* completed its range of action.

The result of the treatment reveals that *Nux vomica, Arsenicum* and *Colocynth,* each had its own curative action but only on the respective parts of the disease course. Though *Arsenicum* matched the symptoms very well after *Nux vomica*, it could not completely remit the case as its action stopped beyond a certain limit of the disease course. It, then, passed over the case to *Colocynth* to complete the recovery like a sporting relay-race. Master Hahnemann, in aphorism 167 to 171, amply suggested such step-by-step treatment with remedies which are most appropriate at different stages of a disease.

11.4 SYNTHESIS

The case further demonstrates that the application of remedies must keep pace with the speed of symptom evolution, whether fast or slow. In an altered state of the disease symptoms, there is a corresponding necessity to change the remedy. In most cases of chronic diseases, a single remedy does not match the entire range of a disease course which possesses many unknown variables including pathology. As a result, a 100% similarity is not obtained in a single remedy. Therefore, the different parts of the disease course are covered by different remedies. It is irrelevant how many remedies are eventually required or how fast the remedies are required to be changed to cure the entire disease course. The speed of symptom evolution may vary from a few minutes to a few hours in acute diseases and from a few days to a few weeks to a few months in chronic diseases. At each stage of the change of symptoms, the remedy needs to be changed to achieve a faster recovery. On the positive side, this is the implication of the speed of symptoms evolution whether in acute or chronic diseases. On the negative side, if the change of a remedy when indicated is not done at appropriate time in a serious acute disease which is of fatal nature, a human life may be lost. Though a single case is too small to draw any gross generalisation of a conclusion, the observations made in the case are valuable and may suggest that such phenomena may exist in many cases.

❖❖❖

CHAPTER-12

Types And Nature Of Medicinal Aggravations

12.1 APHORISM 157 AND 158

Master Hahnemann observed that after ingestion of an appropriate remedy, even if in minute doses, it causes a kind of aggravation of the disease state in the first hour or first few hours. He called it creation of a similar but stronger medicinal disease which subsequently annihilated the natural disease. A slight homoeopathic aggravation during the initial hours is considered as a good prognosis that the disease will yield to the remedy. George Vithoulkas says that there can not be any cure without an aggravation, whether perceptible or imperceptible. But it is not yet clearly known what are various types, nature, duration and controlling factors of homoeopathic aggravation. It is commonly perceived that there will certainly be a great variation in the nature of aggravation because a number of variables would be involved in the process of creation of an aggravation. These may include relative appropriateness, dose, potency and frequency of remedy, nature of disease (acute or chronic), severity of disease, vitality of patient, etc. I cite here three case reports which might indicate the existence of at least three types of homoeopathic aggravations in terms of their duration and other constraints.

12.2 THREE CASE REPORTS

An acute case of a fever in a small boy, Master R, aged 10 years, who was presented on 9th December, 1996, had *Bryonia* symptoms (constipated stool, thirst for water and relief from rest). The remedy was given in three doses of 30C potency, four hourly, and it removed his fever. The process of remedial action in the case was closely monitored. It was found that the first dose of *Bryonia* 30C instantly gave relief to his symptoms for first three to four hours including remission of temperature from 102° F to 100° F. With the second dose given after four hours, the disease aggravation started raising the temperature from 100° F to 103° F. It persisted for about three to four hours. Then, on administration of the third dose after another four hours, the fever started steadily remitting and came down to normal temperature in the next few hours.

In a second case, a middle aged man, Mr. K, aged 47 years, was suffering from intestinal worms for about two months. His symptoms were excessive anal itching in the evening, fetid mouth smell, lot of salivation, frequent appetite, much gas formation and constipated and sour smelling stool. Based on these symptoms, he was given three doses of Cina 30C, four hourly, on 14th December, 1996. The remedy gave him immediate relief which persisted for about two days. After two days, an aggravation of anal itch again started and he became almost restless. He came rushing for further medicine but he was persuaded not to take any more medicine and to bear with the symptoms for some time. Interestingly, after another two to three days the aggravated condition including his anal itch started reducing and he was completely relieved in the next three to four days.

In a third case, a young boy, Mr. D, aged 20 years, was presented on 7th December, 1996, with chronic asthma which had been affecting him for last twelve years. He was on allopathic steroid medicines from time to time. His symptoms were acute respiratory difficulty at times, coughing < 3-4 A.M ; does not like to give out much symptoms about himself (i.e. secretive); fastidious about dresses; likes sweets; controls his temper; father has a history of asthma (i.e. a condition of heredity). Based on these symptoms he was given three doses of *Thuja* 30C four hourly. The remedy gave him considerable relief for about three days but after that a severe aggravation of his asthmatic condition took place for a period of five to six days. Then, again, relief of the symptoms started and continued for the next two weeks.

12.3 ANALYSES OF THE CASES

The above cases when analysed and compared show that the remedial action in all the three cases broadly followed some kind of pattern. The remedy in each case after its administration gave immediate relief of symptoms which varied from a few hours in the acute disease to two to three days in the recent disease and to five to six days in the chronic disease. This stage can be considered as a phase of initial relief which was dynamically a phase of remedial absorption or assimilation by the body. Then, a phase of aggravation which was a reactive phase between the medicine and the body (vital force) followed. This phase continued till the reaction, whether biochemical or in energy form, stopped. The product of this reaction was a curative phase which ensued at the end of the phase of aggravation. Thus, three distinct phases of medicinal actions were recognised during the treatment of acute and chronic diseases. So, it can be inferred that the potentised medicinal actions do follow a particular principle of triphasic activity (fig.1), namely Phase-I (initial relief or assimilation phase), Phase-II (aggravation or reactive phase) and Phase-III (recovery or curative phase).

Next, regarding the duration of each phase it is observed that the initial relief phase (Phase-I) had relatively short duration compared to that of aggravation phase (Phase-II). In acute disease, the initial relief and aggravation phases were only of a few hours while in recent or semi-chronic disease these two phases were spread over a few days. In the case of chronic disease (e.g. third case), the aggravation phase persisted for five to six days which meant that the reaction between the medicine and the body (vital force) continued for a longer period in such disease. Similarly, the curative phase (Phase-III) in the acute disease was very short in the order of only a few hours. In recent disease, it was for a few days while in the chronic disease the curative phase (Phase-III) with 30C potency was in the order of a few weeks which could even be a few months or a few years with higher potencies.

12.4 DISCUSSION

The above-mentioned facts and observations when summarised especially with reference to the aggravation phase (i.e. phase-II), it is found that there could exist at least three types of aggravation pattern. In acute disease, the homoeopathic aggravation would be very short (e.g. three to four hours), in recent or semi-chronic disease it could have ranged from two to three days, while in chronic disease it might spread over six to seven days. Since in the present case reports, one variable of the remedies (i.e. the potency 30C) was constant it can be inferred that the relative chronicity of a disease could be one of the controlling factors towards the duration of reactive phase (i.e. aggravation). It was observed by Dr. J.T. Kent that higher potencies (e.g. 200, 1M, 10M, 50M, CM) had relatively longer curative actions in chronic diseases. But it is not specifically known whether higher potencies had proportionately longer period of initial relief (Phase-I) and aggravation phase (Phase-II) too. It seems unlikely because the speed of assimilation of a medicine and its subsequent reaction would depend upon the urgency of the body's requirement to fight the disease. If a disease is acute, serious, fatal and fast developing in nature, the rate of assimilation of a remedy would accordingly be faster whether in low or high potency. Then, the reactive phase (i.e. aggravation) would also be shorter since the body required to combat such a serious disease quickly enough for its survival. So, the duration of initial relief and aggravation phase would also partly depend upon the severity of a disease. In conclusion, it could emerge that the homoeopathic aggravations (Phase-II) would have at least three time limits of duration depending upon the chronicity and severity of a disease:—

1. Short duration in the order of three to four hours in acute diseases.
2. Moderate duration in the order of two to three days in recent or semi-chronic diseases, and
3. Longer duration in the order of six to seven days in chronic diseases.

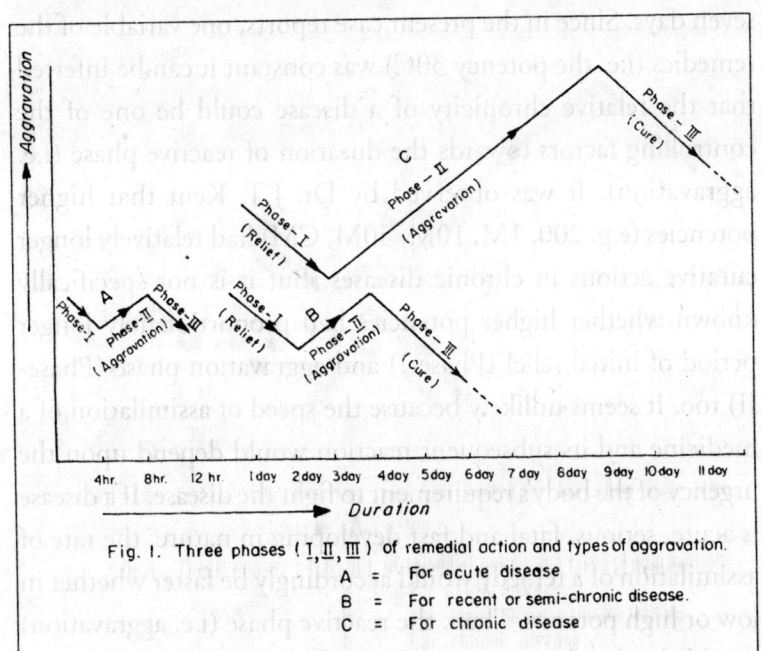

Fig. 1. Three phases (I, II, III) of remedial action and types of aggravation.
A = For acute disease
B = For recent or semi-chronic disease.
C = For chronic disease

CHAPTER - 13

Disease Versus Mind : A Homoeopathic Understanding

In recent times, there have been a series of controversies and debates among the learned homoeopaths regarding the presence of physical diseases vis-a-vis mental states of human beings. One such example is the statement of Dr. Rajan Sankaran who considers " you cannot have a *Sepia* leucorrhoea without a *Sepia* mind". On the other hand, George Vithoulkas states that it is not necessary for a woman with *Sepia* leucorrhoea to have a *Sepia* mind. To look at this basic problem, we first look at what the mastermind of homoeopathy Dr. Samuel Hahnemann says in the *Organon of Medicine*. In aphorism 210, master Hahnemann states that....... "in all corporeal diseases the condition of the disposition and mind is always altered". So, "in all cases of disease we are called on .... the state of the patient's disposition is to be particularly noted along with the totality of symptoms".

From the above statements of Master Hahnemann, it is obvious that the state of the mind of a person is altered during a sickness. In this respect, Dr. Sankaran's statement is justified. But Hahnemann has not said about the degree of alteration of the mind and the temporal status of the alteration, transient or permanent. It may be one of the probable reasons why this point has become debatable. But the change of mind (i.e. mental state) shall be present in a patient in mild, moderate or strong degree depending upon the nature of the disease and sensitivity of the patient. It means that the alteration of mind will always be present during a sickness whether the physician or the patient can perceive it or explain it or not. The alteration can be very incipient, or it may not be externally manifested, or even it may not be perceived by the patient if one is not acutely sensitive. The alteration may even remain at the subconscious level. Unless the alteration of mind is pronounced and peculiar in its manifestation we usually do not consider it in the process of remedy selection. If mental symptoms are not prominent or manifested enough we depend on other characteristic symptoms or essences for the finding simillimum. From this viewpoint Dr. George Vithoulka's statement is also justified.

We need to recognise at the same time two important aspects of the controversial paradigm. One is the "presence of altered state of the mind" and other is the "external manifestation of altered state of the mind" during a sickness. It is obvious that Dr. George Vithoulkas put more stress on the second part of the paradigm while Dr. Rajan Sankaran in his statement gave more stress on the first part of the paradigm which was a two-component entity. So, both the physicians were justified in their own ways of explanation which mainly considered one aspect of the issue. Master Hahnemann considered both aspects of the paradigm. When both sides of the paradigm are considered, there arises no ambiguity. A little rigidity in concepts probably gives rise to such debates. Hahnemann's statements embraced all aspects of the phenomenon of a disease.

Now, is considered the statements of two great exponents of homoeopathy, Dr. George Vithoulkas and Dr. Rajan Sankaran, specifically regarding a *Sepia* leucorrhea from the viewpoints of my experience. What I have observed is that a *Sepia* leucorrhea may develop either in a genetically *Sepia* constitution, or in any other non-*Sepia* constitution. In the former case, we can usually get a *Sepia* mind along with the *Sepia* leucorrhea. But in the latter instance, *Sepia* mind may not develop in all the cases of a *Sepia* leucorrhea but still we can get the remedy *Sepia* based on other characteristic (or peculiar) symptoms which may even be the physicals. Of course, we may not know whether a *Sepia* mind developed in such cases or not incipiently, mildly or subconsciously. According to Dr. Hahnemann, the mind has altered whether we perceive it or not. In this respect, Dr. Sankaran's viewpont is relevant. But we have to select the simillimum based on characteristically manifested symptoms and not on unmanifested symptoms or conceptual situations. For example, a *Sepia* mind with *Sepia* leucorrhea can also develop in a genetically *Arsenicum album* constitution after suffering by the patient for a cause, period and intensity. To develop a mental state (e.g. stasis) like that of Sepia in an active and restless mind like that of *Arsenicum*, the patient must suffer in some *Sepia*-specific ways from the disease and the environment. The *Sepia*-specific ways of the disease evolution (e.g. leucorrhea) is yet to be fully known. This is true for all other non-*Sepia* genetic constitutions. But it is immaterial whether a *Sepia* mind develops or not, or it is perceived or not in all cases of *Sepia* leucorrhea for the purpose of remedy selection which has to be done by all considerations. That is why master Hahnemann stressed on the "*totality of symptoms*" so that one does not falter.

That the state of a mind is altered during a sickness can also be perceived from other examples. For instance, the persons suffering from hypertension (i.e. high blood pressure) usually show a higher degree of mental tension, irritability and anxiety. These mental symptoms are very pronounced in some cases while in some other cases these may not be externally manifested in a prominent way. But they will always remain in incipient, mild or subconscious level in latter category of persons. So, the mental effect of a physical disease only varies in degree, quality, persistence and time. But its creation is unequivocal whether we perceive it or not. However, in certain cases it may be very temporary. Since, a disease is a dynamic phenomenon, its action on human body shall certainly produce some reactions (i.e. effect) to human mind whether transient or long term, mild or strong. Even a temporary acute disease like viral flu creates a mental state like that of *Gelsemium* or *Bryonia* or *Rhus tox.* or *Arsenicum album* whether we can perceive it or not, or a patient can explain it or not. Of course, we can select a simillimum based on the characteristic physicals as well without considering the mentals.

So, there seems to arise no controversy if we consider the following four different parameters which are essential aspects of the paradigm of remedy selection:—

(i) Presence of mental symptoms;

(ii) Characteristic manifestation of mental symptoms;

(iii) Degree of development of mental symptoms (e.g. incipient, mild, moderate and strong);

(iv) Nature of persistence of mental symptoms (e.g. transient, short duration, medium duration, long duration, permanent).

CHAPTER-14

Relative Frequency Of Manifestations Of CDE (Cause-Disease-Effect) Phenomena

During the clinical practices all three types of phenomena (CDE) are encountered from time to time. But can we determine which phenomenon of CDE complex is manifested more frequently than others by the patients? It may be possible to determine statistically their frequency of occurrence if meticulous records are kept by a physician for every case of disease one treats. All cases are to be classified into three categories whether one has prescribed a *cause-based* remedy, a *disease-based* remedy, or an *effect-based* remedy. Sometimes, it is possible that a remedy has been given based on more than one phenomena because two or three phenomena were prominent and have indicated the same remedy. Many a times, it is found that a patient's constitutional remedy is indicated in his disease sphere or effect sphere. In such cases, the simillimum can be called *Hahnemannian simillimum*.

It is often expressed in some quarters that if one peculiar symptom or essence can be picked up, other symptoms of the case fall in line and place. This is not observable very often because the cause, disease and effect symptoms are mostly of different genesis and may not have affinity to the same remedy except in some constitutional selections. For example, in a certain case, the causative remedy may be *Arnica*, the disease remedy may be *Lycopodium* and the effect remedy may be *Acid. nitricum*. Now, the choice for the first remedy to be administered may be different for different physicians. But, in true sense, the choice of the first remedy should be same for all the physicians. However, in clinical practices, this does not always happen because different physicians perceive the symptoms, view the symptoms, consider the symptoms and give weightage to the symptoms in different ways. But standard rules for homoeopathic application say that the treatment should start from the latest symptoms. Besides this, in my experience, it was observed that a treatment could be initiated from any of the following symptoms:—

1. The most prominent symptoms (mental, physical or causal).
2. The symptoms which are most disturbing to the patient's mind.
3. The symptoms which are most focussed by the patient.
4. The symptoms which the patient desires to be treated first.
5. The most troublesome physical symptoms to the patient.

Relative Frequency of Manifestations of CDE Phenomena

6. The most peculiar symptoms related or unrelated to the disease.

7. The symptoms which are clinically gravest to the patient.

It is difficult at present to assess statistically the correct figure of CDE phenomena in terms of their numerical percentage because no such data base and information are available on a larger scale. But, in my experience, some relative assessment could be made about these phenomena. For example, though a causative phenomenon shall be present behind every case of a sickness it is not always determinable in all cases of pathogenic and non-pathogenic events. The patients either cannot recollect such phenomena or correlate such phenomena with their sicknesses in most cases. For pathogenic causes, they are however of no significance in homoeopathic remedy selection except in the cases of nosode remedies. For nosode remedies, the selection is based on miasmatic symptoms. In some cases, the remedies are also based on causative pathogens. For example, *Variolinum* for small pox, *Varicillinum* for chicken pox, *Diphtherinum* for diptheria, *Parotidinum* for mumps. The scope of the use of medicines based on causative pathogens is, however, very limited in homoeopathy. One of the main reasons is that the same pathogens (e.g. bacteria, virus, fungus) can produce different sets of symptoms in different human beings because of their different constitutional and environmental backgrounds.

In overall, thus, the use of causative phenomena in remedy selection is the lowest in terms of numerical statistics. Now, let us consider the status of other two phenomena i.e. D and E. Out of these two events i.e. disease and effect, I could observe that most of the remedies were selected on the basis of disease phenomena. It means that the disease and its related symptoms are manifested more prominently and more frequently than the effect symptoms. Though theoretically, every disease is likely to have some effects on the body and mind, they may not be clearly perceived or differentiated by the patient unless they are very prominent, intense or peculiar. So, there lies the paradox in collecting and evaluating effect phenomena. In analogy of every action having a reaction, the disease being a dynamic phenomenon shall have some reactive phenomena (i.e. effect) on mental and physical spheres of a human being. In practice, however, we are not able to elucidate it (i.e. effect) in every case because of the variously explained reasons. Now, it can emerge that a majority of the remedies are selected on the basis of disease phenomena. It means that the disease symptoms are manifested in most cases in a more frequent, prominent, perceptible and explainable manner. Next frequently used remedies can be considered to be the effect remedies. Therefore, the order of frequency of manifested CDE phenomena and their related remedies can be sequenced in terms of abundance as follows:—

Disease(D) ———> Effect(E) ———> Cause(C)
phenomena   phenomena   phenomena
(Frequent)   (Less frequent) (Occasional)

CHAPTER-15

Relative Importance of CDE Phenomena

15.1 BACKGROUND

It is now well known that the cause, disease and effect (CDE) phenomena are identifiable in all events of human sicknesses. Can we determine which phenomenon is relatively more important in a remedy evaluation and how it is to be determined? Every case of a sickness has its own evolutionary history. It starts with an etiological (causative) background. Then, the disease progresses and affects particular parts of the body, or the whole body, or mind, or emotion. If the entire history of a sickness is analysed, we can split the total sickness phenomenon into three clear-cut components i.e. cause, disease and effect of the disease. Can we define specifically which component is more important? The generalised answer is "No" because any of the components could be significant in a particular case. For instance, if we can determine and relate for sure that a physical injury, recent or remote, is the cause of a particular sickness, then the related injury remedy (e.g. *Arnica, Bellis perennis, Hypericum, Spigelia or Ledum*) can act as a simillimum. The causative remedy becomes more important here for the treatment of this particular case. It is applicable whether the case is acute, recent or chronic. But such cases have also their own limitations.

15.2 LIMITATIONS

A limitation is encountered where the pathology of a disease reached beyond a particular level (i.e. optimum level). For example, when a tumor has developed as a remote effect of an injury and has now turned into a malignancy, the causative remedy does not work here. Then, we try to look for either a disease-based remedy, or an effect-based remedy. Either of these remedies can act as a simillimum. So, the importance of CDE phenomena also depends on the stage of pathological development of a sickness. In this respect, the statement of Dr. J.C. Burnett (1989) is quite relevant. He states that each remedy has its own range of action beyond which the remedy does not work. It was based on his practical observations. What we also observe today is that a remedy does not work beyond a particular pathological level. So, for any remedial (therapeutic) measures we need to keep pace with the stages of disease evolution. The concept of three-component remedial measures (i.e. CDE) possibly matches with the course of a disease evolution, whether in acute, chronic or incurable case. So, individually, any of the three components shall have its own limitations during the treatment of a chronic disease. But the three types of remedies e.g. causative remedy, disease remedy and effect remedy together

Relative Importance Of CDE Phenomena

possibly provide a total remedial response to a disease evolution from its begining to end.

15.3 SOME CASE EXAMPLES

15.3.1 ALLERGIC ITCHING

A lady, aged 35 years, came on 28/03/2000 for treatment of a severe allergic itching in her whole body. It started about five months ago. She took lots of modern anti-allergic and steroid medicines from a skin specialist. She could not remember any causative factor of her ailment. Disease symptoms were not very characteristic. There were no specific modalities for aggravation or amelioration. But she described the following symptoms very poignantly. She told that whenever she got an acute attack of itching she lost her appetite (rubric : Appetite, wanting). She also got poor sleep during the acute stage of an attack (rubric : sleeplessness). She felt sad and morose during and after the acute attack (rubric: sadness, morose). Technically, these symptoms can be called concomitants to the disease. But these are truly the consequences of her main disease (i.e. allergic itching), which were created and felt in other parts of the body and mind following allergy attack. They constitute the effect phenomenon. Based on these effect symptoms she was given one dose of *Sulphur* 200C. It relieved all her symptoms miraculously. Here, the effect phenomenon has overridden all other phenomena in matters of importance in remedy selection.

15.3.2 ECZEMA

A middle aged girl, Ms. S.B., came for treatment of her eczema in both hands and feet. She was in bad condition as lesions tended to suppurate, crack, ooze, bleed, itch from time to time for last five years. It was a kind of allergic manifestation with secondary infection affecting her skin. She was physically weak. She got burning of soles. She was first given *Hepar sulph.* 200C and then *Petroleum* 200C without much benefit. On query to how the disease started and from where it started, she could recollect that the disease first affected her feet and then after one year it spread to her palms. Based on this peculiar symptom movement of the disease, she was given one dose of *Ledum* 200C on 26.10.99. The remedy brought in a dramatic recovery of her eczema in hands and feet. One dose of *Ledum* 200C was working for 5 (five) months with progressive healing of her skin. In this case, a peculiar symptom of the disease led to the simillimum. So, the disease symptom was more important here than the cause or effect symptoms in remedy selection.

15.3.3 EXCESSIVE HAIR FALL

A lady, Mrs. C.K., aged 35 years, came on 06/02/2000 for treatment of her excessice hair fall which started one year ago. She also had hypertension. She was slowly becoming bald. Her scalp was visible at several locations of her head because of the hair fall. She wanted first to stop her hair fall than to cure her hypertension. Her disease and effect symptoms were not much characteristic. Then, I enquired into her constitutional symptoms. She was a hot patient. She liked sweets and salts.

She had burning sensation of soles of feet and vertex of head. She was short-tempered. Her menses were scanty. She had epigastric tenderness. Based on the constitutional symptoms, she was given *Sulphur* 1M/1D. The remedy stopped her hair fall within fifteen days. Then, gradually, new hairs started coming. After two months, a substantial growth of hairs was noted. Hairs thickened and darkened. Here, her constitutional remedy worked as curative. It means that the constitutional susceptibility was the cause of her ailment. So, the causative (i.e. constitutional) remedy was more important than all other remedies in this case of disorder.

15.4 REMARKS

How we decide which of the three types of phenomena (CDE) is to be chosen for a particular sickness? There are several factors in it to be considered. It shall depend upon the clarity, prominence, characteristics, peculiarity (mental and physical) and patient's focus of symptoms. For example, if a patient asserts that his cataract developed after an injury of his eye, the simillimum shall be *Arnica* (high) on causative phenomenon if the pathology has not progressed too far to reach a destructive stage. In some cases where exogenic causative factors are not known, or the disease symptoms or the effect symptoms are not pronounced, then constitutional remedies can be considered. Constitutional susceptibility is an endogenic causative phenomenon. If a constitutional remedy is not workable because his/her constitutional symptoms are not clear, then we may look for a miasmatic remedy, whether inherited or acquired.

Miasmatic susceptibility can also be considered as another endogenic causative phenomenon. In clinical practice, it rarely occurs that we get symptoms equally pronounced, strong and peculiar from all the three spheres of a sickness. Characteristic symptoms or essences are manifested in either one or two spheres and the remedy is selected based on that sphere although we consider all the three spheres in search of characteristic symptoms and the simillimum.

✦✦✦

CHAPTER-16

Epilogue

16.1 In homoeopathy, the fundamental law of cure is *similia similibus curentur*. Master Hahnemann proposed drawing out similarity from the totality of symptoms. This method of finding simillimum is undoubtedly infallible. The principle of similia similibus curentur also opened up several possibilities of working on the simillimum in different spheres of human body and mind. As a result, various learned physicians attempted to work out simillimum in different ways and contexts. Boenninghausen, Kent, Vithoulkas, Jan Scholten, Sankaran and a few others put forward some of the outstanding ideas in this field. Any methodology of finding simillimum if applicable and efficaceous in curing diseases universally is contributory to this system of therapeutics. Even if the innovation of simillimum for a particilar type of disease or for some types of diseases is made possible, it is no less contributory. Works relating to specific disease-oriented simillimums (e.g. cancer, AIDS, heart diseases, Parkinson's, Alzheimer's) can also be attempted for further advancement on specific lines. Such efforts can also lead to the development of specialised fields in homoeopathy. These are no less important for establishing the credibility of this system of therapeutics for handling critical and serious diseases and developing as an alternative therapy to other systems of medicines, particularly the modern medicines which are progressing at a rapid pace.

16.2 An approach towards simillimum based on the *cause, disease and effect phenomena* either singly or in combination is found to be highly efficacious in the treatment of human diseases, acute or chronic. The various case reports as described in previous chapters provide enough testimonials to the efficacy of such an approach if the pathology has not progressed too far to cause destructive changes at the tissue level or molecular changes at the cellular level. Even, in the case of progressed pathology, we have alternatives to search for simillimum. Here, the disease-based or effect-based simillimums can be inducted. We need to filter out and discriminate between the disease symptoms and effect symptoms which are disease-consequences, direct or remote. We can utilise the sphere of symptoms, which has latest, pronounced, peculiar and characteristic symptoms. If both the spheres (i.e. disease and effect) of symptoms are pronounced and peculiar, we can combine them together to work out a simillimum. If one sphere is more pronounced and characteristic than the other sphere, the remedy can be selected from the more pronounced and peculiar sphere.

16.3 I cite here a few acute case reports where the symptoms only from the disease spheres were utilised to find out simillimums. In one case, a young boy aged 16 years had an attack of acute fever on 16/06/2000. He felt very sleepy. His eyes were discharging water. The fever started around 10-11

AM in the morning. Based on these symptoms, he was given *Natrium mur.* 30C/3 doses/4 hourly. It quickly relieved his fever and other complaints. In another case, the disease symptoms changed in quick succession. A man aged 35 years suffered from sudden bouts of vertigo, nausea, vomiting, acidity and restlessness. The sudden feeling of vertigo developed at 9 AM in the morning of 12/06/2000. Severity of the attack made him restless and fearful. He was given *Aconite* 6C/1 dose. After about 15 minutes, the symptoms changed. Now, the vertigo was aggravated from any slightest movement of the body. He was given *Bryonia* 200C/1 dose. He was better for sometime. But after about half an hour, the symptoms changed further. He developed nausea, sour vomiting, excessive gas formation, giddiness and headache. He was immediately given *Lycopodium* 200C/1 dose. He was soon cleared of all his complaints. The medicines were given at the every change of evolving symptoms. So, the use of medicines must keep pace with the stages of evolution of symptoms to bring about quicker relief in some acute diseases, particularly those which are fast progressing and severe in nature.

16.4 The second frequently occurring manifestation of symptoms of a disease occurs in its effect sphere and the simillimum can be selected based on its effect symptoms. I cite here a case of vitiligo in a lady of 28 years of age. She developed a large white spot in the middle of her forehead and top of her feet for last three years. She was in great tension, worry, fear and anxiety about the white spot on the forehead as it was prominently visible (1.5 cm in diameter). The forehead spot appeared later. Constitutionally, she was a *Pulsatilla* patient. But based on her mental effect (e.g. fear, anxiety and worry) of the disease (e.g. vitiligo), she was given *Acid. nitricum* 200C/3 doses/ 72 hourly following Dr. Boenninghausen's principle of dosage interval. After about a month, there was a visible change in the white spot of the forehead. White colour of the skin was getting darker in shade and smaller in size from external margins following Dr. Hering's law of cure. After about two months, a second dose of *Acid. nitricum* 200C was given. It further improved her white spot on the forehead reducing its size and darkening the skin. The case is under follow-up.

16.5 No less important is the causative phenomenon for selection of simillimum. But to establish the degree of reliablility of a causal relationship is important for such a workout. This is vital, more so, for the exogenous causative phenomenon because a patient may not either remember well the causative event or he may provide information which may not be the true causative phenomenon. As a result, the assumption of linking a causative phenomenon can also lead to a wrong diagnosis of a medicine. I cite here a case report which was wrongly diagnosed based on a causative phenomenon as described by the patient. A young girl, aged 19 years, came with a complaint of intermittent breathlessness. She told that she got this problem after an injury of her chest three years ago while travelling in a bus. Based on this information, she was given *Arnica* 200C/3 doses/12 hourly. For 15 days there was no reaction. Then, she was given *Arnica* 1M/2 doses/ 12 hourly. Still there was no reaction. Then, her constitutional symptoms were taken up. She was a hot patient.

She liked sour and extra salt in the diet. She had chronic constipation. She was sentimental. She was introverted. She used to weep after picking up quarrel with her brother. She used to get breathlessness even during sleep. She was given *Natrium mur.* 200C/3 doses/12 hourly. The remedy worked very well. Gradually, she fully recovered from her complaint of breathlessness. So, her constitutional medicine worked here. The constitutional susceptibility seemed to be the cause of her ailment. Here, the endogenous causative factor (i.e. the constitution) was later considered for the selection of simillimum.

16.6 The exogenous cause (e.g. physical injury) which was presumed to be the apparent reason for her ailment led to the wrong selection of a simillimum. So, it is necessary to be cautious about establishing the relationship of exogenous causative factors to any ailment. It may often be misleading for the selection of a simillimum if such phenomenon is made out to be linked to a disease simply on its face value. Like constitutional cause, the miasmatic cause can also be responsible for many of the diseases. Some physicians prefer to call these cases as constitutional block or miasmatic block but I prefer to call them as constitutional susceptibility or miasmatic susceptibility for the creation and continuation of diseases. It is often observed that certain human constitutions are susceptible to certain specific diseases. Similarly, certain miasmatic backgrounds are also susceptible to certain specific diseases. So, we can utilise either the human constitution or the miasm in certain cases to select the simillimum. It is not that in every case we shall look for the miasm in a remedy selection. But in some cases it is necessary to consider the miasmatic susceptibility for remedy selection and permanent cure of a disease. However, it varies from case to case whether the miasmatic remedy shall be the first remedy, the intermittent remedy, or the final remedy after the use of some basic remedies. Besides the miasms and human constitutions, there are also other causative factors which are useful from time to time for remedy selection. For example, a physical suppression (e.g. *Sulphur* for suppression of skin diseases), or an emotional suppression (e.g. *Staphysagria* for suppression of anger, desire, love) can also lead to creation or continuation of some diseases. Another important endogenous causative factor is hormonal change in the human body (e.g. at puberty or menopause) which can also initiate diseases. So, puberty-related medicines (e.g. *Pulsatilla, Belladonna*) and menopause-related medicines (e.g. *Pulsatilla, Conium, Lachesis*) often become useful as causative medicines. Other causative remedies e.g. *Arnica, Bellis perennis, Ledum*, etc., for physical injury and *Opium, Nux vomica, Sulphur*, etc., for abuse of alcohol are already mentioned.

16.7 The cause, disease (sensu stricto) and effect phenomena are three fundamental components of human sicknesses. It is a scientific fact. So, these basic facts need to be recognised by every student of homoeopathy. Master Hahnemann visualised all of these components. So, he was infallible in selection of simillium. We need to investigate into all the three spheres (i.e. cause, disease and effect) of human sicknesses. In the beginning, we do not know where do occur the uncommon, rare, strange and peculiar symptoms of Dr. Hahnemann, or the essences of Dr. Vithoulkas, or the delusions of Dr. Sankaran. Every human sickness can be looked at in a systematised way, searching symptoms from the *'causative sphere'* (including the miasm and

Epilogue

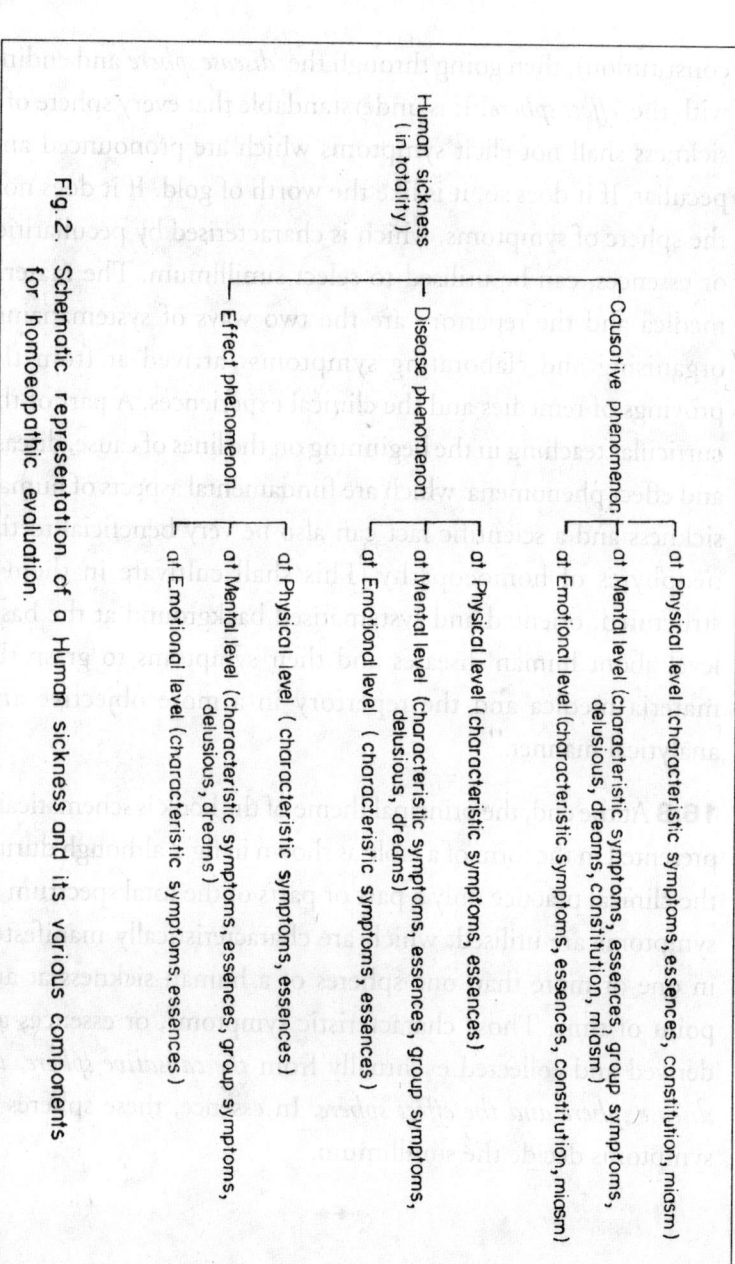

Fig. 2. Schematic representation of a Human sickness and its various components for homoeopathic evaluation.

constitution), then going through the *'disease sphere'* and ending with the *'effect sphere'*. It is understandable that every sphere of a sickness shall not elicit symptoms which are pronounced and peculiar. If it does so, it is like the worth of gold. If it does not, the sphere of symptoms, which is characterised by peculiarities or essences, can be utilised to select simillimum. The materia medica and the repertory are the two ways of systematizing, organising and elaborating symptoms arrived at from the provings of remedies and the clinical experiences. A part of the curricular teaching in the beginning on the lines of cause, disease and effect phenomena which are fundamental aspects of human sickness and a scientific fact can also be very beneficial to the neophytes of homoeopathy. This shall cultivate in them a structured, oriented and systematised background at the basic level about human diseases and their symptoms to grasp the materia medica and the repertory in a more objective and analytical manner.

16.8 At the end, the principal theme of the book is schematically presented in the form of a table as shown in fig.2 although during the clinical practice only a part or parts of the total spectrum of symptoms are utilised, which are characteristically manifested in one or more than one spheres of a human sickness at any point of time. Those characteristic symptoms, or essences are derived and collected eventually from *the causative sphere, the disease sphere and the effect sphere*. In essence, these spheres of symptoms decide the simillimum.

❖❖❖

Bibliography

Alfons Geukens	:	*Inflammation of the middle ear. A case of Silicea. Hom. Links, Vol.13, No. 2-3, 2000.*
Alfons Geukens	:	*Pain in the soles of feet. A case of Silicea. Hom. Links, Vol. 13, No. 2-3, 2000.*
Allen J.H	:	*In cancer and miasmatics by F. J. Bradley. Reprint edition, 1988. B. Jain Publishers (P) Ltd., New Delhi.*
Arora, B.B and Sabarwal, A	:	*Modern's ABC of Biology. Modern Publishers, New Delhi, 1999.*
Barthel, H	:	*Synthetic Repertory(SR), Vol.I&II, Reprint, 1993. B. Jain Publishers (P) Ltd., New Delhi.*
Bradford, T.L	:	*The lesser writings of C.M. Von Boenninghausen. Reprint edition, 1990. B. Jain Publishers (P) Ltd., New Delhi.*
Clarke, J.H	:	*Dictionary of Practical Materia Medica (Vol. I, II, III). Reprint edition,1986. B. Jain Publishers (P) Ltd., New Delhi.*

Cooper, Dorothy, J	: *The nosode Carcinosin. Hom. Update, Vol. 5, No. 9, 1997.*
Darwin, Charles	: *Textbook of Molecular Biology by K.S. Sastry et al, 1994. Macmillan India Ltd., Delhi.*
Dudgeon, R. E	: *The lesser writings of Samuel Hahnemann. Reprint edition, 1990. B. Jain Publishers (P) Ltd., New Delhi.*
Ghegas, Vassilis	: *Conium maculatum: Essence. Hom. Links, Vol. 10, No. 3, 1997.*
Guernsey, W. M. J	: *Desires and aversions. Reprint edition, 1994. B. Jain Publishers (P) Ltd., New Delhi.*
Gypser, K. H.	: *Kent's minor writings on homoeopathy. Reprint edition, 1988. B. Jain Publishers (P) Ltd., New Delhi.*
Hahnemann, S.	: *The chronic diseases. Reprint edition, 1986. B. Jain Publishers (P) Ltd., New Delhi.*
Hahnemann, S.	: *Organon of medicine. Translated by W. Boericke. Reprint edition. 1994. 1986. B. Jain Publishers (P) Ltd., New Delhi.*
Hering, C	: *Analytical repertory of the symptoms of the mind. 2nd reprint edition, 1983. B. Jain Publishers (P) Ltd., New Delhi.*

Hiwat, Corrie and Zee, Harry van der	:	*Interview with George Vithoulkas. Hom. Links, Vol. 13, No. 2-3, 2000.*
Jimenez, Marcos	:	*Carcinosin. Hom. Heritage, Vol.22, 1997.*
Kent, J. T.	:	*Minor writings on Homoeopathy. Compiled and edited by K. H. Gypser. Reprint edition, 1988. B. Jain Publishers (P) Ltd., New Delhi.*
Kent, J. T.	:	*Lectures on Homoeopathic Materia Medica. Reprint edition, 1985. B. Jain Publishers (P) Ltd., New Delhi.*
Kurz, Christian	:	*The last word in homoeopathic posology. Hom. Links, Vol.II, No.1, 1998.*
Mendel, Gregor	:	*Textbook of Molecular Biology by K. S. Sastry et al, 1994. Macmillan India Ltd., Delhi.*
Miller, R.G	:	*Relationship of remedies with duration of action. Repertory of the Materia Medica by J. T. Kent. Reprint edition, 1986. B. Jain Publishers (P) Ltd., New Delhi.*
Nash, E. B	:	*Leaders in Homoeopathic therapeutics. B. Jain Publishers (P) Ltd., New Delhi.*
Payrhuber, Klaus	:	*Two cases with severe pathology. Hom. Links, Vol. II, No. 1, 1998.*
Roy, R. K.	:	*Homoeopathy in cancer treatment. First*

		edition, 2000. B. Jain Publishers (P) Ltd., New Delhi.
Roy, R. K.	:	The symptom movement in Lycopodium. Hom. Links, Vol. 12, No. 4, 1999.
Ortega, P. S.	:	Chronic miasms. Hom. update, vol. 7, No. 2, 1999.
Sastry, K. S. Padmanaban, G Subramanyam, C	:	Textbook of Molecular Biology. Macmillon India Limited, New Delhi, 1994.
Sankaran, R.	:	The spirit of Homoeopathy. Hom.Med. Publishers, Bombay, 1997.
Sankaran, R.	:	Response to interview. Hom. Links, Vol.13, No. 2-3, 2000.
Scholten, Jan	:	Homoeopathy and Minerals. Hom. Med. Publishers, Bombay, 1993.
Scholten, Jan	:	Homoeopathy and the Elements. Hom. Med. publishers, Bombay, 1996.
Scholten, Jan	:	My experience is different. Hom. Links, Vol.13, No. 2-3, 2000.
Steiner, Hansueli	:	The essence of Carcinosinum. Hom. links, Vol. 12, No. 1, 1999.
Tyler, M. and Weir, J	:	Repertorising. Use of repertory by J.T. Kent. Reprint edition,1996, B. Jain Publishers (P) Ltd., New Delhi.

Tyler, M. L.	:	*Homoeopathic Drug Pictures. Reprint edition, 1995. B. Jain Publishers(P) Ltd., New Delhi.*
Vithoulkas, G.	:	*Essence of Materia Medica. Reprint edition, 1994. B.Jain Publishers (P) Ltd., New Delhi.*
Vithoulkas, G	:	*The Science of Homoeopathy. B. Jain Publishers (P) Ltd., New Delhi, 1993.*
Watson, J. D. and Crick, F.H.C	:	*Nature, 171, 1953.*
Whitney, Jerome	:	*The legacy of Rademacher. The Homoeopath, No. 61, 1996.*
Zee, Harry van der	:	*Interview with Alfons Geukens. Hom. Links, Vol. II, No. 2, 1998.*

❖❖❖

You must have enjoyed going through this book. We at **B. JAIN PUBLISHERS (P) LTD.** have many more interesting topics related to this book. Some of them are as follows:—

THE CHRONIC MIASM AND PSEUDO-PSORA
J. H. ALLEN

The title says it all. The book is about the miasmatic theory which was forcefully advocated by Dr. Hahnemann. Very useful for students as well as upcoming Homoeopaths.

BOOK CODE: BA-2006   PAGES: 424   PRICE: Rs. 110.00

CHRONIC DISEASES AND THEORY OF MIASMS
B. JAIN PUBLISHERS

This book is about the diagnosis and treatment of chronic diseases. Also the principles surrounding the miasmatic theory are also dealt with.

BOOK CODE: BB-2091   PAGES: 100   PRICE: Rs. 50.00

HISTORY OF MEDICINE
D. D. BANERJEE

To practice medical profession one has to know the history of the development of medical field which has led to the present know-how.

BOOK CODE: BB-2821   PAGES: 147   PRICE: Rs. 50.00

MIRACLES OF HEALING
ELLIS J. BARKER

Many laymen and doctors are profoundly dissatisfied with orthodox medical method which change from year to year. This book shows the way-out.

BOOK CODE: BB-2044   PAGES: 402   PRICE: Rs. 75.00

B. JAIN PUBLISHERS (P) LTD.
1921, Chuna Mandi, St. 10th Paharganj, New Delhi-110 055
Ph: 3670572, 3670430, 3670572, 3683200, 3683300
Fax: 011-3610471 & 3683400
Website: www.bjainbooks.com, Email: bjain@vsnl.com

You must have enjoyed going through this book. If you want to read more books on Homoeopathy, feel free to write to us and we will rush you a detailed Catalogue.

B. Jain Publishers (P) Ltd.
1921, Chuna Mandi, Street No. 10th, Paharganj,
New Delhi-110 055
☎: 3670430, 3670572, 3683200, 3683300
Fax: 011-3610471 & 3683400
Website: www.bjainbooks.com, Email: bjain@vsnl.com

Subscribe now

HOMOEOPATHIC HERITAGE
(6 issues annually)

A Homoeopathic Journal with a difference

Apart from well researched articles on Homoeopathy, each issue has regulars which include:—

- Editorial by Dr. Farokh J. Master
- Clinical Cases
- Diet and Regimen
- Famous Old Articles
- Book Review
- Homoeopathy Around the World

Chief Editor	: Prof. Dr. Farokh J. Master
Managing Editor	: S. M. Gunavante and Dr. Yogesh Vasandi
House Editor	: Dr. Rohit Jain

For subscription details refer overleaf

B. JAIN PUBLISHERS (P) LTD.
1921, Chuna Mandi, St. 10th Paharganj, New Delhi-110 055
Ph: 3670572, 3670430, 3670572, 3683200, 3683300
Fax: 011-3610471 & 3683400
Website: www.bjainbooks.com, Email: bjain@vsnl.com

Subscription coupon

Yes, I want to subscribe to Homoeopathic Heritage

SUBSCRIPTION RATES FOR ONE YEAR

Overseas in US$	Bangladesh	$ 18/-	India	Rs. 200/-
	Pakistan	$ 32/-	Nepal	
	Rest of the World	$ 40/-	Bhutan	

MODE OF PAYMENT

For India, Nepal & Bhutan by M.O., Bank Draft or Cheque payable at Delhi, New Delhi in favour of **B. Jain Publishers (P) Ltd.**, 1921/10, Chuna Mandi, Paharganj, Post Box 5775, New Delhi - 55, INDIA.

For Overseas by International Money Order or Bank Draft in favour of **B. Jain Publishers Overseas,** 1920, Street No. 10th, Chuna Mandi, Post Box 5775, Paharganj, New Delhi - 110 055, INDIA.

Subscription order form

(Write in Capitals)

Name ....

Complete Mailing Address ....

....

.... Pin ....

Ph. (Res.) .... Ph. (Off.) ....

E-mail. ....

I am remitting Rs./US$ .... by M.O./Bank Draft/Cheque

Date ....   Signature